FRCA: M
the Primary FRCA

C. R. Bailey, F. Moscuzza and A. C. Pearce

FRCA: MCQs for the Primary FRCA

Dr Craig R. Bailey

FRCA

Consultant Anaesthetist
Department of Anaesthesia
Guy's Hospital
London, UK

Dr Franco Moscuzza

FRCA

Consultant Anaesthetist
Department of Anaesthesia
Guy's Hospital
London, UK

Dr Adrian C. Pearce

MRCP FRCA

Consultant Anaesthetist
Department of Anaesthesia
Guy's Hospital
London, UK

W.B. Saunders Company Ltd
London • Philadelphia • Toronto • Sydney • Tokyo

W.B. Saunders Company Ltd	24–28 Oval Road London NW1 7DX, UK
	The Curtis Center Independence Square West Philadelphia, PA 19106-3399, USA
	Harcourt Brace & Company 55 Horner Avenue Toronto, Ontario M8Z 4X6, Canada
	Harcourt Brace & Company, Australia 30–52 Smidmore Street Marrickville, NSW 2204, Australia
	Harcourt Brace & Company, Japan Ichibancho Central Building, 22-1 Ichibancho Chiyoda-ku, Tokyo 102, Japan

A catalogue record for this book is available from the British Library

ISBN 0–7020–2160–1

Typeset by LaserScript, Mitcham, Surrey
Transferred to digital printing 2005

Contents

Foreword

The early years of anaesthetic training have always been burdensome for trainees. In addition to acquiring clinical skills in the broad speciality of anaesthesia, trainees have had to refresh and further develop their knowledge of physiology, pharmacology, physics and clinical measurement and clinical medicine and its interaction with anaesthesia. Since 1996, these subjects have been examined together at one sitting in the Primary FRCA. Candidates therefore need to be able to demonstrate a broad knowledge base during a single examination if they are to progress further in the specialty. This is a daunting task, and it is to the credit of the candidates and their trainers that so many succeed.

MCQs have been used in examinations in medicine for over a quarter of a century to my certain knowledge. At their best they are an effective, efficient and low-cost method of examining a candidate's knowledge, and they are clearly here to stay. Most candidates have some knowledge of them before sitting the primary, but still many have difficulties with the concept. The advice given in the first part of the book is sound and should be read by all, including those with longstanding MCQ experience. After all, it does no harm to remind yourself how to maximise your score!

Standard textbooks give the reader a broad knowledge base, but little insight into how this can be transformed by examiners into MCQ questions. The usual MCQ question books (of which there are many in Anaesthesia) give the answers, usually nothing in the way of explanation. If you disagree or do not understand, back you go to the standard texts and hours of detective work to find the elusive explanation. Craig Bailey, Franco Moscuzza and Adrian Pearce have provided a text that gives the reader the question, the answer and an explanation of the answer, even pointing out that some answers are controversial and discussing the nature of the controversy. As a result, their text is good both for MCQ practice and for learning the revision, and I heartily recommend it.

Rob Feneck
Examiner, Primary FRCA
Anaesthetics Unit, St Thomas's Hospital, London
1998

Introduction

This multiple choice book has arisen from the changes introduced in 1996 to the structure of the FRCA Diploma. This has now reverted from a three-part to a two-part (primary and final) examination in keeping with the changes introduced to specialist training in anaesthesia.

Regulations and Syllabus

The purpose of the primary examination is to assess trainees who have completed a minimum of 12 months' recognized training; they must have limited or full registration with the General Medical Council and registration with the Royal College of Anaesthetists as a postgraduate trainee in the specialty of anaesthesia. It is expected, however, that most trainees will have completed *18 months' training* before attempting the examination. The examination is designed to test:

the candidates' understanding of the fundamentals of clinical anaesthetic practice including equipment and resuscitation;
the candidates' knowledge of the fundamental principles of anatomy, physiology, pharmacology, physics, clinical measurement and statistics as is appropriate for the discipline of anaesthesia;
the candidates' skills and attitudes appropriate to the above level of training.

The examination is in four parts.

Multiple choice questions (MCQs): 90 questions to be completed in 3 hours
physiology and biochemistry (30 questions)
pharmacology (30 questions)
physics and clinical measurement (30 questions).
Objective structured clinical examination (OSCE)
16 stations to be completed in 2 hours.

Viva 1
15 min concerning pharmacology and statistics
15 min concerning physiology and biochemistry.
Viva 2
15 min concerning physics, safety and clinical measurement
15 min concerning clinical topics (including critical incidents).

For detailed information regarding the regulations, syllabus, examination dates and fees, contact:

The Examinations Department
The Royal College of Anaesthetists
48–49 Russell Square
London WC1B 4JY
Telephone 0171 813 1880
Fax 0171 813 1876.

Preparation

MCQs are set because they enable a large cross-section of the syllabus to be covered and are more objective than essays or vivas.

The Royal College have identified two fundamental causes for failure in the examination:

lack of preparation and/or clinical experience with the candidates believing that taking the examination several times is a normal part of the 'training experience';
technical reasons: guessing at MCQs (and therefore accumulating too many negative marks), poor communication skills in the OSCEs and lack of practice for the vivas.

It seems, therefore, that the people most likely to pass the examination are those with a sound knowledge base who organize themselves well; they are in the right frame of mind, and have good time-management and presentation skills.

With regard to obtaining the knowledge required to pass the primary examination it is useful to purchase a selection of core textbooks. Whilst the books may seem expensive they will prove a good investment over time and will be useful not only for the primary but also the final examination. One of the authors (C.R.B.) directed a questionnaire at senior registrars asking them which books and journals they would recommend to trainees preparing for the examination and, based on the results of this survey, we would recommend the books and journals listed at the end of this introduction. If you cannot afford all the books, then buy one large textbook and rely on your departmental library for the remainder. Journals at this stage of your training are useful primarily for their editorial and review articles and we do not recommend ploughing through every article in all the journals listed. Other sources of knowledge include your everyday workload with senior colleagues in the operating theatre, as well as departmental morbidity and mortality, academic and audit meetings. Attending an examination course should provide a good means of revision, but you will gain nothing by listening to lectures on topics which are new to you.

MCQ Technique

Only when you feel that your overall knowledge is adequate should you start attempting MCQs.

When attempting practice papers you may notice a pattern developing early on, for example you answer too few questions, which may indicate that you need to improve your knowledge base; alternatively you may answer most of the questions, but get too many wrong and this usually indicates that your knowledge is faulty or that too many responses are the result of guesswork.

The MCQ paper in the examination consists of negative marking, i.e. a mark is deducted if you answer a question incorrectly; this is to discourage guessing. If people guess every question the probability is that they will score an average mark of zero as half the answers will be correct and half incorrect. However, some people are more successful than others at 'educated guesses' and it is worth, on practice papers, noting as you go along the ones that you are guessing. At the completion of the paper calculate your success rate at guessing; if it is consistently greater than 50%, then guessing some in the actual examination may be to your benefit.

The Examination Paper

The new primary MCQ examination consists of 90 questions, or stems, each question having five parts, or branches, and the time allowed is 3 hours (i.e. 2 minutes per question).

The stem should be read with the branch and constitute a complete sentence that may be true or false. Remember that each option is independent of the others. Read the question carefully;

oxyhaemoglobin may be read mistakenly as carboxyhaemoglobin in the heat of the examination room.

Beware of the following *qualifying words* used in sentences:

'diagnostic', 'essential': must be present for the diagnosis to be made

'characteristic', 'typical': if not present, makes the diagnosis unlikely

'usually', 'commonly', 'frequently', 'majority', 'often': occur in more than 50% of cases

'occurs', 'recognized', 'can be', 'may be': no specific incidence but is reported in most large textbooks on the subject

'rare': < 5%

beware the words 'always' or 'never'; these are usually false as nothing in medicine is absolute!

'approximately': very close to (e.g. the MAC of isoflurane may be quoted as 1.1 in some books but 1.12 in others, and in the examination may be written as 'approximately 1.1').

In the examination we would suggest that you go through the paper answering the questions you are confident of being correct and marking them on the question paper as you go. At the end of this first read through (which should not take too long), read through the paper again concentrating on the questions that you are unsure about but which 'ring a bell'; you should go with your instincts and mark these on the question paper as well. Next transfer all these responses to the computer answer sheet carefully. It is very easy in the heat of the examination situation to fill in the wrong answer on the sheet because one or two questions remain totally unanswered. By now you should still have time available to study the questions which you consider to be very difficult to answer; however, do not dwell on these excessively. It is worth totting up how many answers you have completed; if you have answered 80% then it may not be worth guessing any further answers, but if you have only answered 50% then, assuming that at least a few may be wrong, you must answer more as you are unlikely to pass the examination with a score of 50%.

As soon as you have completed the paper leave the room or you will become neurotic about the questions you initially found straightforward and may end up changing the answer; remember that your initial answer is usually the correct one.

Marking

The completed answer sheets are fed into a computer and an absolute number derived: +1 for a correct answer, −1 for a wrong answer and 0 for an answer left blank or 'don't know'. Therefore a score of between −450 and +450 is obtained.

To be confident of a pass, you should attempt at least 80% of the questions; with the negative marking, this allows you to get 10% wrong but still obtain a final score of 60%, which should see you through.

The results are plotted to obtain a distribution curve. If there is a skew one way or the other, i.e. the particular group of candidates seem to be very good or very bad, then certain 'discriminatory questions' are looked at; these are questions asked in previous years (from a bank of questions). If more candidates answer correctly at this sitting than in previous sittings then it is assumed that the group taking the examination are better overall than in previous examinations and proportionally more candidates will pass.

At this stage some poorly designed questions may be excluded, either because the examiners themselves decide that the answers are ambiguous or that the candidates found the answers ambiguous (half the candidates answered 'true' and half answered 'false', whereas the normal pattern would be a large proportion of candidates giving the correct answer and a smaller proportion answering 'don't know'). If these questions are deleted then a correction will be incorporated into the final score obtained for each candidate.

Candidates are then banded and assigned a grade of 1, 1+, 2 or 2+: 2 or 2+ are passes; 1+ is a bare fail and means that you must obtain a grade 2 or higher in all the other parts to pass the examination overall.

It is interesting to note that the Royal College released information regarding the results of the first sitting of the new primary examination in 1996. There were 141 candidates and the mean score achieved in the MCQ was 53.53% (ranging from a mean of 44% in pharmacology to a mean of 60% in physiology) and only 30.5% of the candidates passed the MCQ (i.e. obtained a score of 2 or better). It should be noted that the examiners were very disappointed in the low mean score in the pharmacology section; this stresses that a candidate cannot pass the MCQ overall if he or she scores a 1 in the individual pharmacology, physiology or clinical measurement sections.

In the primary examination candidates are allowed four attempts; after two failures they are referred to the Bernard Johnson Advisor at the Royal College for guidance.

About the Book

This book contains 360 MCQs arranged as four separate papers of 90 questions similar in format to that found in the examination itself, i.e. a stem followed by five branches, any or all of which may be independently true or false. The first 30 questions concern pharmacology, the next 30 physiology and biochemistry, and the final 30 physics and clinical management. You may wish to attempt a whole paper in one sitting or different sections of a paper at different times. Whilst we have tried to make the questions as unambiguous as possible, there may be some parts of some questions which you find difficult to answer, even if your knowledge is complete; we did not intend to set the questions in this way and apologize for any anxiety we may cause! We hope that although the answers provided are not a substitute for reading textbooks and journals, they do contain substantial amounts of information related to individual questions and should explain most queries that arise. Finally, we should be grateful to receive any comments you would like to make.

Recommended Reading for the Primary FRCA Examination

Text books

A Textbook of Anaesthesia – Aitkenhead, A.R. & Smith, G. (1996) – Churchill Livingstone, Edinburgh.

Ward's Anaesthetic Equipment – Davey, A., Moyle, J.T.B. & Ward, C.S. (1992) – W.B. Saunders, London.

Basic Physics and Measurement – Kenny, G., Davis, P.D. & Parbrook, G.D. (1995) – Butterworth-Heinemann, Oxford.

Essentials of Anaesthetic Equipment – Al-Shaikh, B. & Stacey, S. (1995) – Churchill Livingstone, Edinburgh.

Review of Medical Physiology – Ganong, W.F. (1997) – Appleton Lange, Connecticut.

Respiratory Physiology – West, J.B. (1994) – Williams and Wilkins, London.

Drugs in Anaesthetic Practice – Vickers, M.D., Morgan, M. & Spencer, P.S.J. (1991) – Butterworth-Heinemann, Oxford.

British National Formulary – British Medical Association and the Royal Pharmaceutical Press (1994) – Pharmaceutical Press, London.

Drugs and Anaesthesia – Wood, M. & Wood, A.J.J. (1990) – Williams and Wilkins, Baltimore.

Anatomy for Anaesthetists – Ellis, H. & Feldman, S. (1993) – Blackwell Scientific Publications, Oxford.

Lecture Notes in Clinical Medicine – Rubinstein, D. & Wayne, D. (1991) – Blackwell Scientific Publications, Oxford.

Statistics at Square One – Campbell, M. (1996) – BMJ Books, London.

Revision books

Anaesthesia Databook – Mason, R.A. (1995) – Churchill Livingstone, Edinburgh.

Key Topics in Anaesthesia – Craft, T.M. & Upton, P.M. (1992) – Bios Scientific Publishers, Oxford.

Pharmacology at a Glance – Neal, M. (1997) – Blackwell Science, Oxford.

Journals (editorials and review articles)

Anaesthesia
British Journal of Anaesthesia
Anaesthesia Review
Current Opinion in Anaesthesiology
Recent Advances in Anaesthesia & Analgesia
Drug and Therapeutics Bulletin
British Journal of Hospital Medicine
British Medical Journal
Prescribers Journal
Hospital Update
The Lancet
Adverse Drug Reaction Bulletin
Current Problems in Pharmacovigilance

Acknowledgements

We are grateful for the help provided by the postgraduate students who recently attended the primary FRCA examination day-release course at St Thomas' Hospital, as well as trainee anaesthetists at Guy's Hospital who were guinea-pigs for the questions and raised important queries before most of these questions and answers were put in print.

Paper 1

1. **With regard to cisatracurium:**
   A. it is a constituent isomer of atracurium.
   B. it causes the same amount of histamine release as atracurium.
   C. its duration of action (at equivalent potency) is shorter than atracurium.
   D. it undergoes Hofmann elimination.
   E. no laudanosine is produced when cisatracurium undergoes degradation

2. **Regarding prostaglandins:**
   A. PGD_2 is a bronchodilator.
   B. prostacyclin causes an increase in renin release.
   C. PGE_1 increases gastric mucosal blood flow.
   D. $PGF_{2\alpha}$ causes uterine relaxation.
   E. prostacyclin is a bronchodilator.

1. **AD**

   Atracurium is a mixture of isomers, of which cisatracurium is a single stereoisomer constituent, and represents 15% of atracurium by mass, but has approximately 60% of its relaxant activity, and was introduced into clinical practice on the basis of its pharmacokinetic and pharmacodynamic profiles. The ED_{95} (effective dose required to reduce twitch response by 95% of the control twitch response) is 0.05 mg/kg; a dose of 0.15 mg/kg is recommended to provide good intubating conditions at 2 min and which lasts 55 min. Cisatracurium undergoes non-enzymatic degradation (Hofmann elimination) and very small amounts of laudanosine are produced during degradation. Although there is a little histamine release, this does not appear to be a problem clinically.

2. **BCE**

   There are 14 natural prostaglandins, which are produced from the metabolism of membrane phospholipids:

   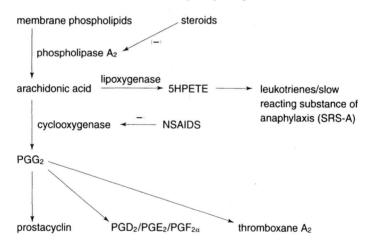

   The main use of prostacyclin (epoprostenol) is as a vasodilator, e.g. in the treatment of pulmonary hypertension and to maintain patency of dialysis machine tubing. The main use of PGE_1 (misoprostol) is to increase gastric mucosal blood flow and also to maintain a patent ductus arteriosus in premature babies. The main use of $PGF_{2\alpha}$ is to stimulate uterine contractions (i.e. induce labour). Both prostacyclin and PGE_1 cause bronchodilation, whilst PGD_2 and $PGF_{2\alpha}$ cause bronchoconstriction.

3. **Clonidine:**
    A. is a β_1-adrenergic agonist.
    B. is administered in low dosage for prophylaxis against migraine attacks.
    C. causes dry mouth as a side effect.
    D. reduces the minimum alveolar concentration of co-administered inhalational agents.
    E. is an anti-hypertensive agent.

4. **The duration of non-depolarizing neuromuscular blockade may be prolonged in the presence of:**
    A. digoxin.
    B. nifedipine.
    C. hyperkalaemia.
    D. chronic phenytoin administration.
    E. fentanyl.

3.   BCDE

Clonidine is an α_2-adrenergic agonist and may be administered orally, intravenously, transdermally and via the epidural route (in a dose of $2\,\mu g/kg$). Clonidine has high bioavailability and a half-life of 9 hours. It is an analgesic (although antanalgesic in very low doses) and acts presynaptically in the peripheral nervous system (reducing noradrenaline release) and post-synaptically in the central nervous system. In low dose, clonidine is used for the treatment of menopausal flushing and for prophylaxis against migraine attacks. It reduces the minimum alveolar concentration of inhalational anaesthetics. Side-effects include dry mouth, sedation, headaches, brady-cardia, nausea, constipation and rash.

4.   BD

Prolongation of action of non-depolarizing neuromuscular blockers may be classified in several ways: by interaction with any part of the pathway from the central nervous system to the skeletal muscle itself; or by classification according to groups of drugs or disorders as shown in the table below.

Drugs

Aminoglycosides

Calcium channel antagonists

Antiarrhythmic agents (procainamide, disopyramide, quinidine)

Inhalational agents

Dantrolene

Chronic phenytoin

Diseases

Myasthenia gravis

Dystrophia myotonica

Endocrine and metabolic abnormalities

Acidosis

Hypokalaemia

Hypocalcaemia

Hypermagnesaemia

Impaired renal function

Liver disease

Hypothermia

5. **Calcium channel blocking agents:**
   A. cause bronchodilation.
   B. are negative inotropic agents.
   C. increase cerebral blood flow.
   D. may precipitate digoxin toxicity.
   E. are used in the treatment of Raynaud's phenomenon.

6. **The following drugs are available in a transdermal preparation:**
   A. fentanyl.
   B. piroxicam.
   C. clonidine.
   D. hyoscine.
   E. buprenorphine.

7. **The principal renal site of action of:**
   A. triamterene is in the ascending limb of the loop of Henlé.
   B. spironolactone is in the descending limb of the loop of Henlé.
   C. frusemide is in the proximal tubule.
   D. osmotic diuretics is in the distal tubule.
   E. thiazide diuretics is in the cortical diluting segment.

5. ABCDE

The most common calcium channel blockers in clinical use are nifedipine, verapamil and diltiazem. Their main uses are in the treatment of angina, cardiac arrhythmias, hypertension and peripheral vasoconstriction (e.g. Raynaud's phenomenon). In general, calcium channel blockers are negative inotropes, increase coronary blood flow and reduce left ventricular end-diastolic pressure, increase cerebral blood flow, increase lower oesophageal sphincter tone, potentiate the side-effects of inhalational anaesthetic agents and cause bronchodilatation. Side-effects include headache, flushing, dizziness, peripheral oedema, an increase in the risk of digoxin toxicity and prolongation of neuromuscular blockade.

6. ACD

Fentanyl, clonidine, hyoscine, glyceryl trinitrate and nicotine are all available in transdermal preparations. The advantages of transdermal administration include ease of use, prolonged duration of action, systemic uptake and avoidance of first pass metabolism in the liver. Buprenorphine is administered sublingually, whilst piroxicam (and other non-steroidal anti-inflammatory drugs, NSAIDs) and eutectic mixture of local anaesthetics (EMLA) cream are topical preparations designed for local absorption rather than systemic uptake.

7. E

Diuretics may be classified according to their mode of action within the kidney. Osmotic diuretics act on the proximal convoluted tubule by producing an osmotic load. Loop diuretics act on the ascending limb of the loop of Henlé; this is impervious to water but chloride is actively reabsorbed and sodium follows electrostatically so that tubular fluid becomes hypotonic. Loop diuretics inhibit chloride reabsorption (and hence sodium) and this creates a lower osmotic gradient between the cortex and medulla so that larger volumes of urine are formed. Thiazide diuretics act on the cortical diluting segment (just proximal to the distal convoluted tubule) of the loop of Henlé by preventing the active reabsorption of sodium which takes place there. Spirono-lactone (an aldosterone antagonist), amiloride and triamterene act on the distal convoluted tubule by reducing sodium reabsorption (in exchange for potassium and hydrogen ions).

8. **Adverse reactions associated with amiodarone include:**
   A. retinal deposits.
   B. pneumonitis.
   C. hypothyroidism.
   D. peripheral neuropathy.
   E. ventricular arrhythmias.

9. **With regard to volatile anaesthetic agents, the rate at which the alveolar concentration approaches the inspired concentration is:**
   A. more rapid for sevoflurane than halothane.
   B. increased by the second gas effect.
   C. increased by increasing alveolar ventilation.
   D. inversely related to the blood:gas partition coefficient of the agent.
   E. decreased by a reduction in cardiac output.

10. **Heparin:**
   A. is a strong acid.
   B. is produced by mast cells.
   C. has a therapeutic half life of 30 min.
   D. may cause thrombocytopenia.
   E. if given for 2 months may cause osteoarthritis.

8. BCDE

Amiodarone has a therapeutic half-life of about 1 month. It is used to treat both supraventricular and ventricular arrhythmias but has many potential adverse effects, including the following:

lung: fibrosis, alveolitis or pneumonitis

liver: abnormal liver function tests, acute hepatitis, fibrosis or cirrhosis

neurological: peripheral neuropathy, or cerebellar dysfunction

eye: corneal microdeposits (noticed as haloes around bright lights) or optic neuritis

thyroid: hyperthyroidism, hypothyroidism or euthyroidism with abnormal thyroid function tests

skin: photosensitivity, rashes, alopecia or dermatitis

heart: prolongation of Q–T interval or bradycardia.

9. ABCD

The rate at which alveolar concentration approaches inspired concentration for a volatile anaesthetic agent is determined by delivery of the agent to the alveoli compared with loss of agent from the alveoli into arterial blood. Input can be increased by: increased alveolar ventilation; increased inspired anaesthetic concentration; the second gas effect; and breathing system characteristics. Loss of agent from the alveolus is increased by: high cardiac output; a high blood:gas partition coefficient; and a high alveolar to mixed venous partial pressure difference.

10. ABD

Heparin, an acid mucopolysaccharide, is one of the strongest natural body acids and is produced by mast cells. Heparin acts by forming a complex with antithrombin III and the activated clotting factors II, IX, X, XI and XII. It has a plasma half-life of 80 min and a half-life effect on clotting of 100 min and is inactivated in the liver (by heparinase) and excreted in the urine. Adverse effects include bleeding, osteoporosis, alopecia and thrombocytopenia.

11. **Regarding suxamethonium (scoline) apnoea:**
    A. it is an autosomal dominant disorder.
    B. a single abnormal cholinesterase gene is found in approximately 4% of the general population.
    C. there are at least four variants of the cholinesterase gene.
    D. dibucaine number is the percentage inhibition of cholinesterase by 10^{-5} M dibucaine (cinchocaine).
    E. normal individuals have a dibucaine number of 100%.

12. **The following drugs cross the placenta in clinically significant amounts when given in conventional dosage during labour:**
    A. intravenous fentanyl.
    B. intravenous neostigmine.
    C. intravenous diazepam.
    D. epidural bupivacaine.
    E. intravenous ketamine.

13. **The following drugs have a low (< 50%) oral bioavailability:**
    A. warfarin.
    B. digoxin.
    C. glyceryl trinitrate.
    D. lignocaine.
    E. aspirin.

11. BD

Suxamethonium apnoea is an autosomal recessive disorder. At least seven variants of the cholinesterase gene have been identified: usual (*u*), atypical (*a*), silent (*s*), fluoride resistant (*f*), H-type, K-type and J-type. Normal people (*Euu*) form approximately 96% of the population and have a dibucaine number of 80 (percentage inhibition of cholinesterase by 10^{-5} M dibucaine). Heterozygotes are apnoeic for 10 min, whilst homozygotes are apnoeic for several hours. The condition is not life-threatening provided it is recognized (this is an important reason why patients given suxamethonium for the first time should have documented evidence of return of neuromuscular function before non-depolarizing drugs are administered, because the combination of drugs may lead to diagnostic confusion and inability to 'reverse' the patient at the end of the procedure); patients with prolonged apnoea should be artificially ventilated (and sedated) until the condition wears off. The patient and their relatives should be investigated at a later date.

Davis, L., Britten, J.J. & Morgan, M. (1997) Cholesterase: its significance in anaesthetic practice. *Anaesthesia* **52**: 244–60.

12. AC

In the placenta, the chorionic villi (the layer of cells that enclose the fetal capillaries) are bathed in maternal blood. This barrier has the same general characteristics as lipid membranes elsewhere in the body, and factors that influence passive passage include the size of molecule (molecular weight < 600 cross easily), percentage plasma protein binding, lipid solubility and ionization. However, there are also active transport mechanisms for sugars, amino acids and vitamins. Finally the placenta contains monoamine oxidase (MAO), cholinesterase and a microsomal enzyme system and is able to metabolize some drugs.

13. CDE

Bioavailability is the proportion (expressed as a percentage) of an administered substance that reaches the systemic circulation. If a drug is administered orally, there are several steps in preventing its appearance in the systemic circulation, of which the most important are lack of absorption and the proportion of first pass metabolism in the liver. Lignocaine, glyceryl trinitrate and aspirin are all extensively metabolized on first passage through the liver and therefore have a low oral bioavailability.

14. **The following have a blood:gas partition coefficient greater than 1:**
    A. halothane.
    B. enflurane.
    C. isoflurane.
    D. sevoflurane.
    E. desflurane.

14. ABC

The following have a blood:gas partition coefficient of greater than 1: halothane, enflurane and isoflurane. The following have a blood:gas partition coefficient less than 1: desflurane, sevoflurane and nitrous oxide. The blood:gas partition coefficient is a useful concept because it implies that an anaesthetic agent with a low coefficient is slowly taken up from the lungs into the bloodstream, allowing target concentrations to build up in the alveoli and hence inducing anaesthesia more quickly as compared with agents having a high coefficient.

	Halothane	Enflurane	Isoflurane	Desflurane	Sevoflurane
Molecular weight	197	184	184	168	200
Boiling point	50.2	56.5	48.5	23.5	58.5
Vapour pressure at 20°C (mmHg)	244	172	240	664	160
Minimum alveolar concentration (MAC)	0.76	1.68	1.15	6	2
Blood:gas solubility	2.5	1.9	1.4	0.42	0.69

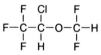

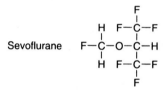

15. **Which of the following statements are correct:**
    A. Zero-order kinetics means that the rate of change of concentration of a drug is independent of that concentration.
    B. First-order kinetics means that the rate of change of concentration of a drug is inversely proportional to that concentration.
    C. A volume of distribution that is greater than the total body fluid volume implies that the drug is concentrated in the tissues.
    D. The plasma half-life is the time taken for half the administered drug to be eliminated from the body.
    E. Clearance is influenced by the volume of distribution at steady state.

15.   AC

Zero-order kinetics means that the rate of change of a drug's concentration is independent of that concentration (i.e. there is saturation), whereas first-order kinetics implies that the rate of change in concentration of a drug is directly dependent on its concentration at the time (and hence an exponential curve is produced).

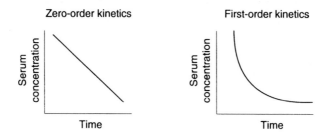

Volume of distribution (V_d) is the volume in which a drug appears to be distributed if it is present throughout the body in the same concentration as that found in plasma. Plasma half-life is the time taken for the plasma drug concentration to fall to half of its initial concentration. Clearance can be envisaged as the volume of plasma cleared of drug in unit time (i.e. ml/kg per min). It is independent of actual volume of distribution.

16. **Administration of hyperbaric oxygen (HBO) therapy is useful following systemic poisoning with:**
    A. paraquat
    B. carbon monoxide.
    C. hydrogen sulphide.
    D. paracetamol.
    E. cyanide.

17. **With regard to cardiac anti-arrhythmic drugs:**
    A. phenytoin causes a prolongation of ventricular repolarization.
    B. bretylium acts as a membrane stabilizer by blocking sodium channels.
    C. flecainide is effective in both ventricular and supraventricular dysrhythmias.
    D. calcium channel blockers are effective for supraventricular tachydysrhythmias.
    E. lignocaine is effective for both ventricular and supraventricular dysrhythmias.

16. BCE

HBO administration is under-utilized in the UK despite the fact that it is of proven value in many disease states and following drug toxicity. Among the published conditions in which HBO has been successfully used are the following:

> air and gas emboli
> decompression sickness
> wounds (clostridia and tetanus)
> burns
> toxins (carbon monoxide, hydrogen sulphide, cyanide)
> rheumatic conditions (systemic lupus erythematosus and scleroderma)
> radiation necrosis
> necrotizing fasciitis
> refractory osteomyelitis.

HBO therapy may have the following effects: inhibition of the actions of cytokines; providing an excess of dissolved oxygen; increasing the clearance of toxins; enhancing wound healing by causing fibroblast and capillary proliferation; and reducing local oedema.

17. CD

Anti-arrhythmic agents are traditionally divided into four classes (as described by Singh and Vaughan Williams) depending on their mechanism of action. Class I agents are membrane stabilisers and include lignocaine, mexilitine, quinidine, flecainide and phenytoin, whilst Class II agents include the β adrenergic blockers, Class III bretylium and amiodarone and Class IV the calcium channel blockers.

18. **Appropriate antibiotic cover for adult patients with a prosthetic heart valve undergoing dental work under general anaesthesia:**
    A. gentamicin alone.
    B. amoxycillin plus gentamicin.
    C. vancomycin plus gentamicin if there is penicillin allergy.
    D. flucloxacillin alone.
    E. teicoplanin.

18. BC

The British Society for Antimicrobial Chemotherapy has recommended the following prophylaxis for adult patients requiring general anaesthesia.

Heart murmur

Amoxycillin 3 g orally preoperatively or 1 g i.v. at induction of anaesthesia plus 500 mg 6 hours later

Prosthetic heart valve or previous infective endocarditis

Amoxycillin 1 g i.v. plus gentamicin 120 mg i.v. at induction

Penicillin allergy or penicillin within the last month

Vancomycin 1 g i.v. at induction plus gentamicin as above, or

Teicoplanin 400 mg i.v. at induction plus gentamicin, or

Clindamycin 300 mg i.v. at induction plus 150 mg orally 6 hours postoperatively

---

Working Party of the British Society for Antimicrobial Chemotherapy (1992) Antibiotic prophylaxis of infective endocarditis. *Lancet* **339**, 1292–3.

19. **The following drugs are contraindicated in patients with acute intermittent porphyria:**
    A. propofol.
    B. etomidate.
    C. thiopentone.
    D. ketamine.
    E. halothane.

20. **With regard to the following agents which act on the sympathetic nervous system:**
    A. ephedrine is both an α and β agonist.
    B. yohimbine is an α_1 agonist.
    C. phentolamine is a pure α antagonist.
    D. metaraminol is an α antagonist.
    E. prazosin is an α_1 antagonist.

19. BC

The porphyrias are a group of inherited disorders due to defects in the metabolism of porphyrins (which form coordination complexes with various metals, such as iron in haemoglobin). The severe form of porphyria, acute intermittent porphyria (AIP), is an autosomal recessive disorder most commonly found in South Africans, from where most of the anaesthetic literature is derived. AIP is important as it commonly presents with lesions in the central and peripheral nervous systems, and attacks can be precipitated by drugs and can resemble an abdominal emergency. Unsafe drugs include the barbiturates, sulphonamides, steroids and etomidate. Local anaesthetics are safe to give but may cause a change in the neurological status of the patient, who should be warned about this. The following drugs are considered safe:

    opioids
    ketamine
    propofol
    inhalational anaesthetic agents
    suxamethonium
    non-depolarizing neuromuscular blocking agents
    atropine
    neostigmine.

Vickers, M.D., Jones, R.M. (eds) (1989) Genetics and inherited disease. In *Medicine for Anaesthetists*, 3rd edn, pp. 327–49. Blackwell Scientific Publications, London.

20. ACE

α and β receptors
+ adrenaline, ephedrine
− labetalol

α receptors
+ noradrenaline, metaraminol
− phentolamine

β receptors
+ isoprenaline
− propranolol

α_1	α_2	β_1	β_2
+ phenylephrine	+ clonidine	+ tazolol	+ salbutamol
− prazosin	− yohimbine	− atenolol	− butoxamine

21. **Hyoscine:**
    A. has a longer duration of action than atropine.
    B. is a more potent antisialogogue than atropine.
    C. may cause a fever.
    D. is a superior antiemetic compared with atropine.
    E. causes more tachycardia compared with atropine.

22. **Droperidol:**
    A. is a thioxanthine.
    B. increases cerebral blood flow.
    C. is antiemetic in large doses only.
    D. may cause hypotension.
    E. is metabolized in the liver.

23. **Morphine:**
    A. is vagotonic.
    B. may cause spasm of the sphincter of Oddi.
    C. reduces release of antidiuretic hormone (ADH).
    D. causes pupillary constriction.
    E. is a pure μ-receptor agonist.

21. ABCD

Hyoscine is an anticholinergic agent that crosses the blood–brain barrier. Compared with atropine 0.6 mg, hyoscine 0.4 mg has a prolonged duration of action, causes less tachycardia, is a more effective drying agent and is a superior antiemetic. It is also a bronchodilator but may cause central nervous system depression. Like other anticholinergic agents, hyoscine can cause fever, constipation, pupillary dilatation and urinary retention.

22. DE

Droperidol is a butyrophenone similar to haloperidol. It acts on several different receptors (including α adrenergic and dopamine); whilst it is antiemetic in very low doses, α adrenergic blockade may result in hypotension and it is a psychomotor tranquillizer. Droperidol reduces cerebral blood flow and its clinical effects last approximately 8 hours. Compared with phenothiazines, droperidol causes less hypotension, sedation and anticholinergic side-effects but its potential adverse effects include dysphoria and extrapyramidal signs.

23. ABD

Morphine is a natural product of the opium poppy. Opiate receptors have been located in the spinal cord (periaqueductal grey matter), the substantia gelatinosa and the medial thalamic nuclei. Clinical effects of morphine include the following; in the central nervous system morphine causes analgesia, depression of respiration and the cough reflex, stimulation of vomiting (via the chemoreceptor trigger zone), stimulation of Edinger–Westphal nucleus and convulsions. In the cardiovascular system, morphine causes bradycardia, hypotension and vasodilatation. Other effects of morphine include sphincter spasm (Oddi and urinary), pruritus, histamine release and increase in secretion of ADH. Opioid receptor subtypes have been identified as shown in the table.

Receptor	Effect of stimulation	Agonist	Antagonist
μ_1	Analgesia	Morphine	Naloxone Nalorphine
μ_2	Respiratory depression Pupillary constriction	Morphine	Naloxone Nalorphine
δ	Reduction in the sympathetic response to hypovolaemia	Enkephalins	Naloxone
κ	Sedation	Dynorphins Morphine	Naloxone
σ	Dysphoria	Dynorphins	Naloxone

24. **The following are true regarding sucralfate:**
    A. it contains aluminium.
    B. it helps to prevent gastric, but not duodenal, ulcers.
    C. it is given once daily.
    D. it is safe in patients with renal failure.
    E. it is cheaper than ranitidine.

25. **Effects of dopamine include:**
    A. blunting of the hypoxic drive.
    B. increase in systemic vascular resistance.
    C. increase in aldosterone concentration.
    D. increase in cardiac output.
    E. increase in heart rate.

24. AE

Sucralfate protects the gastric and duodenal mucosa from ulceration, and contains aluminium hydroxide and sulphated sucrose. The drug is only minimally absorbed and the small amount is excreted renally. Its use is not recommended in patients with severe renal failure due to the risk of aluminium toxicity. It is administered in a dose of 2 g twice a day or 1 g four times a day, and costs 35p per day. This compares with cimetidine 61p per day, ranitidine 93p per day and omeprazole £1.27 per day.

25 ABDE

Dopamine is a natural inotropic agent with specific receptors in the kidney and mesenteric blood vessels. In low dose (up to $2.5 \mu g/kg$ per min) dopamine acts on dopamine receptors only, resulting in an increase in renal blood flow; in progressively higher concentrations it has agonist effects on first β_1-adrenergic ($2-5 \mu g/kg$ per min) and then α-adrenergic ($> 5 \mu g/kg$ per min) receptors. However, there is great overlap in these effects and significant individual variation; even at low doses dopamine may increase cardiac contractility and systemic vascular resistance. Renal effects of dopamine may result from a combination of the following: increase in cardiac output, local effects on dopamine receptors increasing renal blood flow, reduction in aldosterone secretion and a direct effect on renal tubular function. There has been a recent backlash on the use of renal-dose dopamine for the maintenance of renal blood flow because of the following negative aspects of dopamine:

tachycardia;
blunting of the hypoxic ventilatory drive;
gut ischaemia: in experimental animals there is a reduction in oxygen extraction in the mesenteric circulation possibly due to precapillary vasoconstriction with diversion of blood away from the gut mucosa – this redistribution causes a decrease in oxygen extraction despite increased blood flow;
reduced gastric motility;
increased metabolic rate;
increase in endocrine and immune dysfunction, with reduced secretion of growth hormone and prolactin.

Thompson, B.T. Cockrill, B.A. (1994) Renal dose dopamine: a Siren song? *Lancet* **344**, 7–8.
Cuthbertson, B.H., Noble, D.W. (1996) Dopamine in oliguria. *BMJ* **314**, 690–1.

26. **For a given whole blood drug concentration, factors influencing the rate of passive diffusion of drug molecules across a capillary membrane include:**
    A. molecular size.
    B. ionization of molecule.
    C. lipid solubility.
    D. Bunsen solubility coefficient.
    E. percentage plasma protein binding.

27. **Free hepatic intrinsic clearance is:**
    A. always much higher than measured hepatic clearance.
    B. influenced by red cell penetration by the drug.
    C. influenced by protein binding.
    D. the hepatic clearance divided by (1 − the extraction ratio).
    E. higher for thiopentone than methohexitone.

28. **With regard to the ionization of acids and bases:**
    A. weak bases have a $pK_a > 7.4$.
    B. weak acids in solution cannot exist in alkaline pH.
    C. the concentration of the ionized form of weak bases increases with an increase in pH.
    D. increasing the H^+ concentration decreases the ionized form of weak acids.
    E. strong acids are highly ionized at pH 7.4.

29. **The following drugs, in therapeutic dosage, have the described approximate percentage plasma protein binding:**
    A. morphine, 40%.
    B. thiopentone, 80%.
    C. pancuronium, 50%.
    D. diazepam, 75%.
    E. fentanyl, 85%.

26. ABCE

Protein binding is important because it is only the unbound fraction of the drug that is diffusible. Unionized, lipid-soluble molecules up to a molecular weight of 600 pass relatively easily. The Bunsen coefficient relates to gas solubility, i.e. the volume of gas dissolving in unit volume of liquid at standard temperature and pressure (STP).

27. D

Actual or measured hepatic clearance of a drug is influenced by factors such as protein binding, hepatic blood flow and red cell penetration, because these factors affect the amount of free drug at the site of metabolism. Free intrinsic clearance is not influenced by these factors and is a calculated measure of clearance of unlimited, unbound drug at the site of metabolism. It is the measured hepatic clearance corrected for extraction ratio (the higher the extraction ratio, the higher the intrinsic clearance). The value for thiopentone is 4 ml/kg per min and for methohexitone is 23 ml/kg per min.

28. DE

Acids are proton donors and bases are proton acceptors. A weak base (B) accepts a proton (H^+) to become charged (BH^+) and the concentration of BH^+ will increase with a fall in pH.

$$Base + H^+ \longrightarrow BaseH^+$$
$$Acid \longrightarrow Acid^- + H^+$$

The pK_a is the pH at which there are equal concentrations of charged and uncharged base or acid. Diazepam is a weak base (pK_a 3), whilst thiopentone is a weak acid (pK_a 7.9).

29. ABE

Most acidic drugs are bound to albumin, whereas basic drugs are often bound to other proteins such as α_1-acid glycoprotein. In general, protein binding correlates with lipid solubility (although this correlation is not true for ketamine, which is highly lipid soluble yet only 12% bound to plasma proteins). The value for diazepam is very high at 99%. The values for the ionized muscle relaxants are low: pancuronium and vecuronium are 30% and atracurium is 50%. When plasma protein binding is high, small changes in binding will produce a great change in the percentage of free drug.

30. **Non-competitive drug interactions include:**
    A. benzodiazepines and γ-amino butyric acid (GABA).
    B. protamine and heparin.
    C. guanethidine and phenylephrine.
    D. α-bungarotoxin and nicotine.
    E. bretylium and noradrenaline.

31. **The following conditions cause an abnormally increased bleeding time:**
    A. massive blood transfusion.
    B. haemophilia A.
    C. von Willebrand's disease.
    D. vitamin K deficiency.
    E. disseminated intravascular coagulation.

32. **Platelets:**
    A. are formed in the spleen from megakaryocytes.
    B. circulate for approximately 1 month.
    C. may be labelled with radioactive iodine.
    D. contain heparin-neutralizing substances.
    E. contain 5-hydroxytryptamine (serotonin).

30. ABCDE

A competitive drug interaction is when drugs compete for the
same receptor site (e.g. morphine and naloxone), whereas a
non-competitive drug interaction is any other form of interaction. Benzodiazepines enhance the effects of GABA, an
inhibitory neurotransmitter. Heparin activates antithrombin III
and protamine neutralizes the action of heparin. Guanethidine
is selectively taken up into adrenergic nerve endings and
accumulates in noradrenaline storage vesicles from which it is
released in response to nerve impulse, whereas phenylephrine
acts mainly by a direct action on the adrenergic receptor.

31. ACE

The bleeding time depends principally on platelet number,
function and platelet–capillary interaction, not whole blood
clotting. The traditional Ivy method involves inflating a
tourniquet around the upper limb to 40 mmHg and timing
the flow of blood from cuts 1 cm long and 1 mm deep on the
forearm. The upper limit of normal is 7 min. Aspirin leads to
irreversible acetylation of platelet cyclooxygenase, rendering it
inactive. Von Willebrand's disease is an autosomal dominant
condition characterized by abnormal bleeding and elevated
prothrombin and bleeding times. Disseminated intravascular
coagulation is the widespread intravascular deposition of fibrin
with consumption of clotting factors and platelets.

32. DE

Platelets are round or oval discs 2–4 μm in diameter, formed in the
bone marrow from megakaryocytes. At any one time 80% of
platelets are found in the circulation and 20% are found in the
spleen. The half-life of platelets is 7 days. Radiolabelling of small
venous thrombi is accomplished by labelling fibrinogen, not the
platelets themselves. Platelets aggregate at the site of injury and
release the contents of their granules. One type of granule contains
adenosine diphosphate (ADP) and serotonin. The ADP promotes
platelet stickiness and further granular release. Phospholipase A_2
in the platelet membrane causes release of arachidonic acid from
membrane phospholipids, which is converted to prostaglandins
and thromboxanes including thromboxane A_2. These substances
cause further aggregation and release. Prostacyclin (PGI_2) is
produced in endothelial cells and inhibits aggregation.

33. **With regard to the central venous pressure waveform:**
    A. the *a* wave is due to atrial filling.
    B. no *a* wave is visible in atrial fibrillation.
    C. the *c* wave is increased in tricuspid regurgitation.
    D. pressure values are increased with chronic obstructive pulmonary disease.
    E. pressure values are reduced in cardiac tamponade.

34. **A mixed venous oxygen saturation measurement of 55% may be due to:**
    A. general anaesthesia itself.
    B. hypovolaemia.
    C. hypothermia.
    D. sepsis.
    E. cardiac failure.

33. BCD

The *a* wave occurs during atrial systole (because some blood regurgitates into the superior vena cava) and is absent in atrial fibrillation (and atrial flutter). In complete heart block and nodal rhythm, contraction of the right atrium against a closed tricuspid valve produces a giant *a* wave (cannon wave) that is regular in nodal rhythm and irregular in complete heart block. The *a* wave is also increased in amplitude in tricuspid stenosis. The *c* wave is a transmitted manifestation of the rise in atrial pressure produced by bulging of the tricuspid valve into the right atrium during isovolumetric ventricular contraction; in tricuspid valve regurgitation, ventricular systole produces substantial retrograde flow into the atrium and superior vena cava, producing a large *c* wave. The *v* wave is due to the rise in right atrial pressure before the tricuspid valve opens. The central venous pressure is increased in cardiac tamponade, right ventricular failure, superior vena caval obstruction and chronic obstructive pulmonary disease. (See diagram for Paper 2, question 31)

34. BDE

The normal arterial–venous oxygen difference is 5 ml/100 ml blood, derived from an average whole body oxygen consumption of 250 ml/min and cardiac output of 5000 ml/min. The normal mixed venous oxygen saturation is approximately 75%. If the value is lower, it indicates that oxygen delivery to the tissues is inadequate for tissue needs; this may be due to reduced oxygen delivery or excessive oxygen consumption. General anaesthesia may reduce oxygen delivery but the low metabolic rate (which is also seen in hypothermia) means that supply is probably in excess of demand. Any process that reduces oxygen delivery (hypoxaemia, low cardiac output, anaemia) will cause a fall in mixed venous saturation that will be even greater if tissue extraction is high, for example in sepsis.

35. The following are true regarding thyroid hormones:
   A. they stimulate hepatic glycogenolysis.
   B. they stimulate absorption of carbohydrates from the gastrointestinal tract.
   C. at high blood levels they stimulate protein synthesis.
   D. the fetus depends on placental transfer of thyroid hormones.
   E. triiodothyronine (T_3) has a half-life of 6–7 days.

35. AB

Thyroxine (T_4) and T_3 are the principal hormones secreted by the thyroid gland. Thyroid hormone secretion is regulated by thyroid-stimulating hormone (TSH) from the anterior pituitary, which in turn is modulated by thyrotrophin-releasing hormone (TRH) from the hypothalamus. Thyroid hormones also exert negative feedback on the pituitary gland. T_3 is the more biologically active agent and has a half-life of about 1 day compared with the 6 or 7 days of T_4. Virtually all (>99%) of the hormone is bound to plasma proteins, predominantly to thyroxine-binding globulin, and it is only the unbound fraction that is active. Thyroid hormones have the following actions:

increase oxygen consumption and heat production;

increase glucose mobilization and plasma glucose concentrations by glycogenolysis;

promote protein synthesis at low levels (but protein catabolism occurs at the high levels seen in thyrotoxicosis);

effects on skeletal growth and development: in the fetus the thyroid is active by approximately the 10th week of gestation and there is negligible transplacental transfer; thyroxine is also necessary for the normal development of the central nervous system;

potentiation of the effects of catecholamines on the cardiovascular system.

36. **The following are true regarding calcium homeostasis:**
    A. active vitamin D causes increased absorption of calcium from the gastrointestinal tract.
    B. active vitamin D causes increased bone deposition.
    C. hypocalcaemia stimulates parathyroid hormone secretion.
    D. parathyroid hormone increases renal calcium reabsorption.
    E. serum calcium is approximately 50% bound to albumin.

37. **With regard to cerebrospinal fluid (CSF):**
    A. normal specific gravity is between 1.003 and 1.009.
    B. approximately 2000 ml is formed per day.
    C. the rate of formation is increased if the intracranial pressure rises.
    D. it is alkaline relative to normal blood pH.
    E. the pressure normally alters with respiration.

36. ACDE

Of total body calcium 99% is found in bone; of the remaining 1% found in the plasma approximately 50% is unionized, bound to albumin and inactive, and the remainder is ionized, free and active. Measurement of serum calcium levels is usually of total calcium (i.e. bound and unbound calcium) and a correction needs to be made for albumin levels (0.02 mmol per gram of albumin above or below 44 g/L). In addition, liberation of free ionized calcium is decreased as the pH is increased (causing the clinical effect of tetany during hysterical hyperventilation for example) and binding of calcium is decreased as pH decreases. Control of calcium levels is achieved by three substances.

> Parathyroid hormone: this is a peptide released by the parathyroid gland and causes an increase in free calcium by stimulating osteoclastic activity, increasing the production of active vitamin D in the kidney and increasing urinary reabsorption of calcium.
>
> Active vitamin D: this is produced in the kidney by conversion of 25-hydroxycholecalciferol to 1,25-dihydroxycholecalciferol and increases calcium absorption from the gastrointestinal tract and increased reabsorption of calcium in the kidney.
>
> Calcitonin: this is a peptide released by the C (follicular) cells of the thyroid gland. Calcitonin reduces gastrointestinal absorption of calcium, reduces resorption from bone and reduces renal reabsorption.

37. AE

CSF is formed in the choroid plexuses (found in the roofs of the third, fourth and lateral ventricles) by a combination of filtration, active transport and diffusion. It has a pH of 7.31 (specific gravity 1.003–1.009) with glucose and potassium concentrations 30–40% lower than in plasma. Total volume is 150–200 ml with daily production being about 600 ml (i.e. there is a complete turnover of CSF three times a day). The normal CSF pressure is less than 15 mmHg and, if transduced, shows a respiratory swing. The rate of formation is independent of pressure up to a value well above the normal lumbar pressure of 180 cm H_2O. The rate of reabsorption by arachnoid villi is proportional to pressure and ceases when the lumbar pressure falls below 70 cm H_2O. The buoyancy of the brain in the CSF gives rise to a net brain weight of only 50 g.

38. **With regard to the eye:**
    A. the normal intraocular pressure is 20–30 mmHg.
    B. the intraocular pressure rises during halothane anaesthesia (assuming normocarbia).
    C. mannitol reduces the volume of the aqueous humour.
    D. topical anticholinesterases cause pupil constriction.
    E. the afferent loop of the oculocardiac reflex is via the optic nerve.

39. **With regard to the control of breathing:**
    A. peripheral chemoreceptors are located in the carotid and aortic arch bodies.
    B. peripheral chemoreceptors respond only to changes in arterial oxygen tension.
    C. central chemoreceptors are located in the pons.
    D. J receptors are situated in the lungs.
    E. the Hering–Breuer inflation reflex is an increase in the duration of expiration produced by steady lung inflation.

38. D

The normal intraocular pressure (IOP) is between 10 and 15 mmHg and values above 25 mmHg are considered pathological. The pressure is primarily due to the balance between production and drainage of aqueous humour, although other factors include choroidal blood volume, vitreous humour volume and external pressure on the eye. Halothane produces a dose-dependent reduction in IOP. The aqueous humour volume may be reduced by acetazolamide, whilst the normal vitreous humour volume of 5 ml may be reduced by osmotic agents such as mannitol. Ocular manipulation may produce a sinus bradycardia (the oculocardiac reflex of Aschner), the afferent limb of which is the ophthalmic division of the trigeminal nerve and the efferent limb being the vagus nerve.

39. ADE

The carotid bodies have the highest blood flow per gram of tissue of all the body organs – 2000 ml/100 g per min or approximately 40 times the cerebral blood flow. The high flow allows a response to falls in oxygen tension rather than oxygen content; they also respond to alterations in hydrogen ion concentration and carbon dioxide tension, and denervation of both carotid bodies abolishes the ventilatory response to hypoxia. Each carotid and aortic arch body contains islands of cells. Glomus cells are closely associated with cup-like endings of the glossopharyngeal afferent nerves and have granules that contain catecholamines including dopamine which are released in response to a reduction in oxygen tension. The central chemoreceptors are located in the medulla on the ventral surface of the brainstem near, but separate from, the respiratory centre and are stimulated by CSF hydrogen ion concentrations. J receptors appear to be stimulated by hyperinflation of the lung and the usual reflex response is apnoea followed by rapid breathing, bradycardia and hypotension.

40. The following cause pulmonary arteriolar vasoconstriction:
   A. angiotensin II.
   B. acetylcholine.
   C. thromboxane A_2.
   D. prostacyclin.
   E. noradrenaline.

41. With regard to total body water:
   A. inulin is used to estimate total body water.
   B. one-third is intracellular.
   C. red blood cells contain 3% of total body water.
   D. Evans blue may be used to directly measure the interstitial fluid volume.
   E. plasma water is approximately 4% of total body water.

40. ACE

The pulmonary vascular system is a low pressure 'distensible' system. Normal systolic/diastolic pressures are approximately 24/9 mmHg. The volume of blood in the pulmonary vessels is 1000 ml. Pulmonary vessels have a sympathetic vasoconstrictor supply but are also responsive to chemicals and oxygen tension. The substances listed in the table cause constriction or dilatation of the pulmonary vasculature.

Vasoconstriction	Vasodilatation
Thromboxanes	Isoprenaline
Adrenaline	Prostacyclin
Noradrenaline	Acetylcholine
Angiotensin II	Oxygen
Carbon dioxide	Nitric oxide

41. CE

Total body water in a typical adult is 45 l, 15 l of which is extracellular and 30 l intracellular. The interstitial fluid is part of the extracellular fluid and cannot be measured directly, although it can be estimated by subtracting plasma volume from extracellular volume. Evans blue is highly protein bound and remains in the intravascular space, allowing measurement of plasma volume (3 l). Inulin, mannitol and sucrose have all been used to measure extracellular fluid volume. Total body water is usually measured with deuterium oxide.

42. Glucagon:
   A. is lipolytic.
   B. stimulates the release of insulin.
   C. has a half-life of 5–10 min.
   D. secretion is stimulated by exercise.
   E. secretion is inhibited by high serum glucose levels.

42.   ABCDE

Glucagon is a polypeptide consisting of 29 amino acids that is synthesized and released by the A cells of the pancreas (and the gastric mucosa). It has a half-life of 5–10 min and has the following main actions:

> liver glycogenolysis and gluconeogenesis are promoted
> lipolysis is promoted
> insulin secretion and ketogenesis are increased
> catecholamine release is increased
> a direct positive inotropic effect on the heart occurs.

The factors listed in the table affect glucagon secretion.

Increase	Decrease
Acetylcholine	Somatostatin
β-Adrenergic agonists	α-Adrenergic agonists
Cortisol	Glucose
Theophylline	Insulin
Stress/exercise/starvation	Free fatty acids/ketones
Gastrin	Secretin

43. **In an adult with 50% body surface thermal burns:**
    A. full thickness burns cause severe pain.
    B. there is a reduction in cardiac output.
    C. antacids should be avoided.
    D. antibiotics should be withheld until a bacteriological diagnosis has been made.
    E. a urinary catheter should be avoided due to the risk of introducing infection.

43. B

Partial thickness burns cause severe pain because pain sensors are still present, but full thickness burns destroy these sensors and so there is little pain or bleeding. Wallace's 'rule of nines' describes a relatively easy and quick way of assessing burn area whereby the head accounts for 9%, the arms 18%, the legs 36%, the torso 36% and the perineum 1%. The table shows the damage that may occur in burns injuries.

Respiratory

Direct damage due to smoke inhalation; damage to cilia, impaired mucus production, mucosal oedema and surfactant depression.

Indirect damage due to systemic absorption of carbon monoxide; increase in carboxyhaemoglobin levels (whose half-life is 4 hours, but may be reduced to 40 min if high-dose oxygen is administered) and cyanide toxicity (> 20 mmol/l).

There is also an increased risk of respiratory infection, wheeze and acute respiratory distress syndrome.

Cardiovascular

Impaired cardiac output due to hypovolaemia, negative inotropic effect of carbon monoxide and a depression factor released systemically following severe burns.

Endocrine and metabolic

There is a risk of myoglobinaemia and myoglobinuria and a urinary catheter should be placed aseptically.

There is a risk of peptic ulceration ('Curling's ulcer') and prophylaxis should be administered.

Tetanus toxoid booster should be given as well as adequate analgesia.

Fluid replacement may follow the Mount Vernon regimen:

$$\frac{\text{body weight} \times \text{estimated percentage burn area}}{2}$$

This volume (in ml) should be given as a mixture of crystalloid and colloid every 4 hours for 12 hours, then every 6 hours for 12 hours, then 12-hourly from the time of injury.

44. **Cerebral blood flow:**
    A. is approximately 15% of the cardiac output.
    B. is directly proportional to the partial pressure of arterial carbon dioxide between 3 and 8 kPa.
    C. is equal to the mean arterial blood pressure less the intracranial pressure.
    D. increases during a grand mal convulsion.
    E. increases with advancing age.

45. **ECG changes associated with hypokalaemia include:**
    A. reduced P-wave height.
    B. shortened P–R interval.
    C. prolonged QRS complexes.
    D. S–T segment depression.
    E. inverted T waves.

44. ABD

Cerebral blood flow constitutes 14% of cardiac output and 18% of total body oxygen consumption. Two-thirds of the blood flow is supplied by the carotid arteries and one-third by the vertebral arteries. Cerebral blood flow depends on the following.

> Cerebral perfusion pressure: this is the difference between mean arterial pressure and the sum of intracranial pressure (due to brain, blood and CSF) and venous pressure (which is normally zero at the jugular venous bulb). Between a mean arterial blood pressure of 60 and 140 mmHg the cerebral blood flow remains constant due to autoregulation.
>
> Partial pressure of arterial carbon dioxide: cerebral blood flow is directly proportional to this value between 3 and 8 kPa.
>
> Partial pressure of arterial oxygen: cerebral blood flow is independent of this unless the value drops to less than 6.5 kPa, when the cerebral blood flow will increase steeply.
>
> Cerebral metabolic rate: if the metabolic rate increases, for example during a convulsion, then cerebral blood flow will increase.
>
> Temperature: increase will result in an increase in cerebral blood flow.
>
> Age: increase in patient age leads to a reduction in cerebral blood flow.

45. DE

The changes shown in the table occur with progressive increase or decrease in serum potassium levels.

Hyperkalaemia	Hypokalaemia
Tall T waves	Prominent U waves
Reduced R-wave amplitude	Small, then inverted T waves
Prolonged QRS complexes	S–T segment depression
Reduced P-wave amplitude	Increase in P–R interval
Sine wave	Ventricular ectopics
Asystole	Ventricular fibrillation

46. **In the assessment and treatment of postoperative pain:**
    A. there is wide interindividual variation in analgesic requirements.
    B. pain scoring systems provide little useful information.
    C. the correct dose of morphine may be easily predicted from the patient's body weight.
    D. cultural and psychological factors play little part.
    E. intermittent intramuscular injections lead to a high incidence of patient dissatisfaction.

47. **Physiological changes in pregnancy include:**
    A. increase in systolic arterial blood pressure.
    B. reduction in serum levels of clotting factors.
    C. increase in oxygen consumption.
    D. increase in functional residual capacity (FRC) of the lungs.
    E. reduction in glomerular filtration rate.

46.   AE

Postoperative pain is a complex subject with a large number of factors, including cultural and psychological, playing a part. Intermittent intramuscular injections lead to a high degree of dissatisfaction and patient-controlled analgesia has a number of advantages including less fluctuation in plasma opioid concentrations, better matching of dose for individual variability and the advantage obtained by restoring patient autonomy.

47.   C

Physiological changes in pregnancy may be classified according to the effects on different organ systems;

Cardiovascular: increased heart rate, reduction in systemic vascular resistance, normal blood pressure, venous engorgement of the epidural space.

Respiratory: increased tidal volume, increased respiratory rate, reduction in FRC.

Renal: increase in renal blood flow and glomerular filtration rate.

Haematological: increase in red blood cell count and proportionally greater increase in plasma volume, resulting in a reduction in haemoglobin concentration, reduction in platelet numbers and increase in clotting factors.

Gastrointestinal tract: increased gastric acid secretion, reduction in lower oesophageal sphincter tone and reduction in the rate of gastric emptying.

Endocrine and metabolic: reduction in albumin, increase in globulin fraction, increase in cortisol and aldosterone secretion.

48. **Compared with normal patients, obese patients:**
    A. are more likely to suffer from postoperative deep vein thrombosis.
    B. require greater volumes of epidural drugs.
    C. have increased chest wall compliance.
    D. have reduced systemic vascular resistance.
    E. may suffer from obstructive sleep apnoea.

49. **Features of spinal 'shock' following high spinal cord transection include:**
    A. spasticity.
    B. bradycardia.
    C. overflow urinary incontinence.
    D. excessive sweating.
    E. hypertension.

48. AE

The following are potential problems involved in anaesthetizing obese patients.

> Airway: large neck, reduced thyromental distance and excess fatty tissue make tracheal intubation potentially difficult.

> Respiratory: reduced chest wall compliance, reduced FRC and increased work of breathing.

> Circulatory: increase in systemic vascular resistance, increased incidence of ischaemic heart disease, hypertension and deep vein thrombosis; venous engorgement of the epidural space (relatively smaller amounts of local anaesthetics required).

> Gastrointestinal tract: increase in intra-abdominal pressure, reduced stomach emptying and increased incidence of hiatus hernia.

> General: difficulty with positioning of the patient, applying monitoring and obtaining venous access.

49. BC

Spinal shock is the condition that develops shortly after spinal cord transection and may last from several hours to several weeks. There is flaccidity with reduced or absent tendon reflexes, passive filling of the bladder and overflow urinary incontinence, and inability to mount autonomic responses leading to hypotension, hypothermia and bradycardia. After this initial phase spasticity develops and autonomic surges in response to stimulation occur, resulting in excessive sweating, hypertension and tachycardia.

50. **Patients who smoke cigarettes:**
    A. are more likely to suffer from hypertension.
    B. have increased levels of ADH.
    C. have increased neutrophil chemotaxis.
    D. have levels of carboxyhaemoglobin up to 15%.
    E. regain normal respiratory cilia activity 24 hours after cessation of smoking.

51. **When considering a patient in the lateral position undergoing one-lung ventilation of the dependent lung:**
    A. blood flow to the dependent lung increases.
    B. ventilation–perfusion mismatch occurs in the dependent lung.
    C. hypoxic pulmonary vasoconstriction occurs immediately in the non-ventilated lung.
    D. ventilation–perfusion mismatch (shunting) in the upper lung is less severe if the lung is already severely diseased.
    E. hypoxaemia is improved by increasing the inspired oxygen concentration.

50. **ABD**

Apart from the long-term hazards of smoking such as ischaemic heart disease, obstructive lung disease and lung carcinoma, smoking has the following adverse effects.

Cardiovascular: nicotine is a positive inotropic agent, causing an increase in heart rate, systemic vascular resistance and blood pressure, whilst inhalation of carbon monoxide results in carboxyhaemoglobin levels of up to 15%, reducing the oxygen-carrying capacity of haemoglobin. These effects may be reduced by cessation of smoking for even as short a period as 24 hours.

Respiratory: increase in mucus production and reduction in ciliary activity which will start to recover 6 weeks after cessation of smoking

Infective: the risk of infections is increased because there are abnormal pulmonary alveolar macrophages (PAMs), a reduction in neutrophil leucocytosis and a reduction in immunoglobulin concentrations and killer T-cell activity, all of which improve within 6 weeks of cessation of smoking.

51. **ABDE**

Blood flow to the dependent lung increases because pulmonary artery pressures are low enough for regional flow in the lungs to be affected by gravitational forces and ventilation to the lower lung is normal. In the unventilated lung there is still blood flow and so a shunt occurs; hypoxic pulmonary vasoconstriction takes some time to occur (and this physiological reponse is impaired if inhalational anaesthetic agents are used or there is hypocarbia). If the oxygen saturations are low with one-lung anaesthesia, the following options should be considered:

increase F_{IO_2}
add positive end-expiratory pressure (PEEP) to the dependent lung
insufflate oxygen to the collapsed lung
clamp the pulmonary artery to the collapsed lung.

52. **Renal blood flow increases in the following conditions:**
    A. exercise.
    B. on standing.
    C. fever.
    D. systemic hypotension.
    E. increased prostaglandin levels.

53. **On rapid mountain ascent to high altitude:**
    A. atmospheric pressure reduces linearly.
    B. there is compensatory hypoventilation to conserve energy.
    C. cardiac output is reduced.
    D. levels of 2,3-diphosphoglycerate (2,3-DPG) increase.
    E. pulmonary oedema may develop.

54. **The following cause a metabolic acidosis:**
    A. aspirin overdosage.
    B. renal failure.
    C. ethylene glycol poisoning.
    D. pyloric stenosis.
    E. ammonium chloride infusion.

52.   CE

Renal blood flow is 1.2–1.3 l/min or approximately 25% of total cardiac output; 75% of renal blood flow is distributed to the renal cortex. The factors listed in the table increase or decrease renal blood flow.

Vasodilatation	Vasoconstriction
Pyrogens	Angiotensin II
Proteins	Hypotension
Prostaglandins	ADH
Parasympathetic stimulation	Sympathetic stimulation
	Serotonin
	Exercise
	Hypoxia

53.   E

Atmospheric pressure does not reduce linearly with altitude because the density of air varies with altitude. When breathing air at altitude, the concentration stays the same but the partial pressures are reduced so that alveolar oxygen tension falls and arterial oxygen saturation declines. Typical values for atmospheric oxygen are: sea level, 21 kPa; 5000 feet, 17 kPa; 10 000 feet, 14.5 kPa. The fall in oxygen tension stimulates peripheral chemoreceptors and hyperventilation occurs, producing a respiratory alkalosis. The cardiac output rises to maintain oxygen delivery to the tissues and there is a slow adaptive increase in levels of 2,3-DPG, which shift the oxygen–haemoglobin dissociation curve to the right. Hypoxia may result in acute pulmonary hypertension and oedema.

54.   ABCE

An acidosis is a strain on the buffering system that would produce a fall in pH of the blood (acidaemia) if it was not compensated. A metabolic acidosis is caused by either increased production or decreased elimination of fixed or 'non-respiratory' acid. The factors listed in the table cause metabolic acidosis.

Normal chloride levels	Increased chloride levels
Ketoacidosis	Renal tubular acidosis
Lactic acidosis	Acetazolamide therapy
Renal failure	Ureteric transplantation into the colon
Aspirin, alcohol or antifreeze overdose	Ammonium chloride

55. **Effects of PEEP may include:**
    A. increase in renal blood flow.
    B. increase in intracranial pressure.
    C. reduction in venous return.
    D. increase in left ventricular end-diastolic volume (LVEDV).
    E. reduction in hypoxic pulmonary vasoconstriction.

56. **A plasma sodium of 110 mmol/l:**
    A. is incompatible with life.
    B. is always treated with twice normal strength (1.8%) saline solutions.
    C. may be due to carcinoma of the lung.
    D. may occur in Addison's disease.
    E. may occur in diabetes insipidus.

57. **Erythropoietin:**
    A. is secreted by the bone marrow.
    B. is a glycoprotein.
    C. has a circulating half-life of 5 days.
    D. is only detectable in the plasma of anaemic patients.
    E. is produced commercially from rat kidneys.

55. BCE

PEEP reduces venous return to the heart and may cause a reduction in both total cardiac output and in regional organ flow.

Advantages of PEEP	Disadvantages of PEEP
Increase in FRC	Increase in pulmonary vascular resistance
Reduction in shunt	Interventricular septal shift causing decrease in LVEDV
	Raised intracranial pressure
	Decreased renal blood flow
	Increased dead space
	Reduced hypoxic pulmonary vasoconstriction.

56. CD

The normal plasma sodium concentration is 132–147 mmol/l; levels of 110 mmol/l are very low and carry a substantial mortality, but are not always fatal. In one study, the mortality of female patients was higher than males. Hyponatraemia may be caused by the following:

excessive free water: polydipsia, syndrome of inappropriate ADH secretion (SIADH), dextrose fluids, high dose oxytocin
loss of salt: diarrhoea, vomiting, diabetes, diuretics
excessive free water and salt, but relatively more water than salt: congestive cardiac failure, cirrhosis, nephrotic syndrome.

The mainstay of treatment is restriction of free water intake and the plasma sodium must not be altered too rapidly. However, in the presence of neurological signs, cautious administration of 1.8% saline to elevate the value to 118–120 mmol/l may be indicated. In SIADH, water restriction may be the only require-ment. In diabetes insipidus, there is vasopressin deficiency and free water clearance is high, leading to hypernatraemia.

57. B

Erythropoietin is a glycoprotein of molecular weight 30 400, released by the peritubular cells of the kidney in response to tissue hypoxia. The active molecule contains 166 amino acids, has a half-life of 4–12 hours and can be measured in the plasma of all patients. It stimulates differentiation of the immature progenitor cell into an adult erythrocyte by acting as a mitosis stimulating factor and differentiation hormone. It is prepared commercially by a recombinant DNA technique.

58. **With regard to histamine:**
    A. three receptor subtypes have been identified.
    B. both H_1 and H_2 receptors mediate vasodilatation.
    C. H_2 receptors in the heart mediate slowing of atrioventricular conduction.
    D. skin generally has H_1 receptors.
    E. it acts via G protein-coupled receptors.

59. **The following are true with regard to compliance:**
    A. it is a change in volume per unit change in pressure.
    B. it is the reciprocal of elastance.
    C. lung compliance depends on surface tension forces.
    D. chest wall compliance depends on elastic recoil.
    E. total compliance is the sum of chest wall and lung compliances.

60. **Myocardial contractility is increased by:**
    A. atropine.
    B. isoprenaline.
    C. raised end-diastolic pressure.
    D. an increase in heart rate from 70 to 140 beats/min.
    E. reduced arterial pH from 7.4 to 7.3.

58. ABDE

Three distinct histamine receptors have now been identified and all act via G protein-coupled receptors, although the second messenger systems are different. Both H_1 and H_2 receptors mediate vasodilatation and this is primarily via vascular endothelium (H_1) and smooth muscle cells (H_2). In the heart, the majority of effects, such as an increase in the force of contraction, heart rate and automaticity, are mediated via H_2 receptors but the direct slowing of atrioventricular conduction is an H_1 receptor effect. The major bronchial effect (bronchoconstriction) is mediated via H_1 receptors but some H_2 receptor-mediated bronchodilation may occur because H_2 receptor blockade can cause bronchoconstriction. The role of H_3-receptor antagonists has not been elucidated.

59. ABCD

Compliance is volume change per unit pressure change and is the reciprocal of elastance.

Lung compliance (typically $200 \, ml/cmH_2O$ or $2 \, l/kPa$) depends on elastic forces, mainly from surface tension (and hence surfactant) and elastic tissue within the lung substance, and varies with lung volume. Chest wall compliance depends mainly on the elastic recoil of the chest wall and is also $2 \, l/kPa$. The compliances of lungs and chest wall are in series (electrical analogy) and the reciprocal of total compliance is equal to the sum of the reciprocal of lung and chest wall compliances.

$$\frac{1}{\text{Total compliance}} = \frac{1}{\text{Lung compliance}} + \frac{1}{\text{Chest wall compliance}} = \text{Elastance}$$

60. B

Myocardial contractility can be increased by increasing the stretch of myocardial fibres at the end of ventricular diastole or by altering the inotropy of the heart. A raised end-diastolic pressure does not necessarily indicate a raised end-diastolic volume and it is ventricular volume that produces fibre stretch. Isoprenaline is a positive inotrope but atropine has no inotropic activity.

61. When considering humidity:

A. relative humidity is the humidity of the inspired gas relative to environmental humidity.

B. the absolute humidity of fully saturated inspired air at 37°C and atmospheric pressure is approximately $44\,g/m^3$.

C. if the temperature of a gas is increased the relative humidity will fall.

D. operating theatre humidity should be kept between 50 and 70%.

E. increased humidity in the operating theatre increases the risks of sparks from static electricity.

62. Laminar flow of a fluid through a tube is:

A. inversely proportional to the density of the fluid.

B. inversely proportional to the length of the tube.

C. directly proportional to the square of the radius of the tube.

D. directly proportional to the pressure difference across the tube.

E. directly proportional to the viscosity of the fluid.

61. BCD

Absolute humidity is the amount of water vapour in a given volume of air (g/m^3) at a given temperature and pressure, whereas relative humidity is the absolute humidity divided by the maximum amount possible if the air were fully saturated with water vapour at that same temperature and pressure and is expressed as a percentage. The maximum possible water content increases with increasing temperature. If a gas is heated, the absolute humidity stays the same but the relative humidity falls. In the alveolus at $37°C$ the absolute humidity is $44 \, g/m^3$ or 100% relative humidity. In the operating theatre the humidity should be kept between 50 and 70%. If the humidity is too high it becomes uncomfortable for the staff, whereas low humidity increases the risk of static electricity and sparks developing.

62. BD

The Hagen–Poiseuille law states that under conditions of laminar flow the flow of a fluid through a tube is described by:

$$\frac{\pi r^4 (P_1 - P_2)}{8\sigma l}$$

where r is the radius, $P_1 - P_2$ the pressure drop, σ the viscosity of the fluid and l the length of the tube. Reynolds number is used to predict turbulent flow. If the number is greater than 2000 then turbulent flow is likely. Reynolds number equals:

$$\frac{vpd}{\sigma}$$

where v is the linear velocity, p the density of the fluid, d the diameter of the tube and σ the viscosity of the fluid.

63. **The following relate to the gas laws:**
    A. Boyle's law states that at constant temperature (T) the volume (V) of a gas varies with its absolute pressure (P).
    B. Charles' law states that at a constant volume (V) the absolute pressure (P) of a gas varies with its temperature.
    C. the combined gas laws state that $PV = kT$ (where k is a constant).
    D. according to Dalton's law of partial pressure, the pressure exerted by each gas in a mixture of gases is the same as if it alone occupied the container.
    E. in a cylinder of compressed air at 100 bar the pressure exerted by oxygen is equal to 79 bar.

64. **Oxygen:**
    A. is flammable.
    B. was first discovered in 1672 by Black.
    C. is often measured in clinical practice by an infrared analyser.
    D. has a boiling point of $-118°C$.
    E. is stored in cylinders at a pressure of 135 bar.

63. ACD

The gas laws may be defined as follows.

> Boyle's law states that, at constant temperature (*T*), the volume of a gas (*V*) is inversely proportional to the pressure (*P*): $V \propto 1/P$.

> Charles' law states that, at constant pressure (*P*), the volume of a gas (*V*) is directly proportional to the temperature (*T*): $V \propto T$.

> Gay-Lussac's law states that, at constant volume (*V*), the pressure (*P*) is directly proportional to the temperature (*T*): $P \propto T$

> This leads to the combined gas law: $PV = kT$, where *k* is a constant.

If air is at 100 bar pressure, then nitrogen is at 79 bar pressure and oxygen at 21 bar pressure.

64. E

Oxygen is a colourless odourless gas that supports combustion, but is not itself flammable. It was discovered in 1777 by Joseph Priestley and is produced commercially by fractional distillation of liquid air. Oxygen may be measured by mass spectrometry, paramagnetic analysers, fuel cells or a Clark electrode. Infrared analysers only function for gases that have three atoms or two different atoms within the molecule.

	oxygen	nitrous oxide	entonox	carbon dioxide
physical state in cylinder	gas	liquid	gas	liquid
boiling point (°C)	−183	−89		−78.5
critical temperature (°C)	−118	36.5		31
critical pressure (atm)	50	72		73
pressure when full (atm)	135	44	135	49

65. **The amount of a gas dissolved in a liquid:**
    A. increases as the temperature of the liquid is increased.
    B. is proportional to the molecular weight of the gas.
    C. is proportional to the pressure of gas above the liquid.
    D. is reduced by the presence of other dissolved gases.
    E. has the same partial pressure as the gas above the liquid at equilibrium.

66. **Regarding critical temperature:**
    A. the critical temperature of a gas is the temperature above which no amount of pressure will liquefy it.
    B. the critical temperature of nitrous oxide is 36.5°C.
    C. above the critical temperature a substance exists as a vapour.
    D. if Entonox is stored below its critical (pseudocritical) temperature it will initially deliver a hypoxic mixture.
    E. the critical temperature of oxygen is −118°C.

65.   CE

Henry's law states that, at a given temperature, the amount of gas dissolved in a liquid is directly proportional to the partial pressure of the gas in equilibrium with that liquid. The concentration of dissolved gas equals the partial pressure of the gas multiplied by its solubility coefficient. As the temperature rises the amount of dissolved gas decreases (remember warm lager is less fizzy!). Dalton's law states that the pressure exerted by a gas at a given temperature is dependent only on that temperature and is independent of the pressure exerted by any other gases occupying the same space. In a mixture of gases the pressure is the same as if each gas alone occupied the space separately and the total pressure is the sum of the constituents. The solubility coefficient is the volume of gas dissolved in a unit volume of liquid; if this is under conditions of standard temperature and pressure it is known as the Bunsen solubility coefficient. If it is measured at the temperature concerned it is the Otswald solubility coefficient.

66.   ABE

The critical temperature is the temperature above which a gas cannot be converted to a liquid by any amount of pressure. Below the critical temperature the substance may exist as a liquid, a vapour or a mixture of both. The relationship between pressure and volume is usually displayed as an isotherm at a given temperature. The critical pressure is the pressure required to liquefy a substance at its critical temperature.

The critical temperature and pressure of one substance may be affected by another; for example Entonox, a mixture of 50% oxygen and 50% nitrous oxide, is stored in cylinders as a gas at a pressure of 137 bar because of the effect of the admixture of the two gases. This is known as the Poynting or overpressure effect. The critical temperature of the nitrous oxide in the mixture also changes from 36.5°C to a 'pseudocritical' temperature of −6°C. Therefore, if cylinders of Entonox are stored below this temperature the nitrous oxide will exist as a liquid and initially pure oxygen is released from the cylinder. Once the cylinder is empty of oxygen the nitrous oxide will vaporize and a hypoxic mixture delivered. (See table in Paper 1, question 64.)

67. The following are true of Mapleson D breathing systems:
  A. they are efficient for spontaneous ventilation.
  B. their physical properties are not affected by the length of tubing.
  C. the Lack system is an example.
  D. some rebreathing occurs at standard fresh gas flows.
  E. during controlled ventilation more rebreathing will occur at faster respiratory rates leading to an increase in end-tidal carbon dioxide concentration.

67. BD

The Mapleson D breathing system has fresh gas delivered directly to the patient end of the system and an expiratory hose, at the end of which is a reservoir (rebreathing) bag with an adjustable pressure limiting (APL) valve. The Bain system is one such example with a coaxial design, the fresh gas being delivered by the narrow internal tube and the expiratory gases being carried in the outer part of the hose. Some rebreathing occurs with these systems at standard fresh gas flows and this can be adjusted by altering the fresh gas flow. It is an inefficient system for spontaneous ventilation as the fresh gas flow required to prevent rebreathing is two to four times the patient's minute ventilation, whilst it is very efficient for controlled ventilation with a theoretical minimum fresh gas flow equal to the patient's minute volume. The bag may be replaced by an automatic ventilator of the bag squeezer type with the APL valve completely closed; in this situation the patient's end-tidal carbon dioxide level is controlled by adjustments to the fresh gas flow, increasing or decreasing the amount of rebreathing, and not by changing the respiratory rate or the tidal volume. The Lack system is an example of a coaxial Mapleson A breathing system.

68. The following are true regarding soda lime:
- A. it contains mainly sodium hydroxide.
- B. for efficient use 25% of the volume of the canister should be space between granules.
- C. it should have a moisture content of approximately 15–20%.
- D. its temperature may rise to 60°C.
- E. it must not be used in a circle system with sevoflurane.

68. CD

Soda lime is composed of 80% calcium hydroxide ($Ca[OH]_2$), 5% sodium hydroxide and approximately 15% water content, in addition to an indicator dye; 1% potassium hydroxide and silicates were formerly added but are no longer thought to be necessary. The reactions are as follows:

$$CO_2 + H_2O \rightarrow H^+ + HCO_3^-$$
$$Ca(OH)_2 + H^+ + HCO_3^- \rightarrow CaCO_3 + 2H_2O$$

These reactions produce heat and also result in a change in pH, which activates the indicator dye. The size of the granules is important and the optimal size is between 1.5 and 5 mm in diameter, which corresponds to a Mesh size of 4–8 (this is the number of lines per inch); if the granules are too fine then the resistance to breathing is high, but if the granules are too coarse then channelling of gases between the granules occurs. Soda lime is capable of absorbing 25 l of cardon dioxide per 100 g but is caustic to the respiratory tract; care should be taken not to overfill canisters and there should be at least 1 m of tubing between the soda lime canister and the patient. The temperature of soda lime increases with use and if it gets too high there is reduced efficiency and increased resistance. Sevoflurane is degraded by soda lime to compound A but not in clinically significant amounts and there are no reports of adverse effects; however it is recommended that fresh gas flows of at least 2 l are maintained in a circle system when using sevoflurane.

69. **With circle absorber systems:**
   A. a minimum fresh gas flow rate of 1 litre is essential.
   B. if a vaporizer in circle (VIC) is used, vaporizer settings usually need to be increased above the desired concentration.
   C. two unidirectional valves are essential.
   D. inspired oxygen concentrations should be monitored only at the common gas outlet.
   E. with the vaporizer outside the circle (VOC) at low flows, rapid adjustments can be made to inspired vapour concentrations.

69. C

Circle systems have an inspiratory and expiratory limb each with a unidirectional valve, a carbon dioxide absorber, a fresh gas source, reservoir bag and APL valve. The vaporizer may be located either in the circle (VIC) or more commonly outside the circle (VOC). There is a large reservoir within the system that will dilute anaesthetic gases at the beginning of anaesthesia and it is usual practice to flush out air at the beginning of a case by providing a high fresh gas flow of anaesthetic agents for the first 5–10 min before reducing the flows in a stepwise manner to the required flows. At low fresh gas flows the oxygen concentration is diluted by the exhaled gases and may be considerably lower than that delivered by the fresh gas, so monitoring of the oxygen concentration actually delivered to the patient is imperative. Vaporizer output will be affected by the fresh gas flow through it. With a VIC, at low flows the vapour concentration will be higher than that dialled up because of both recirculation of gas already carrying vapour and increased saturation of the gas passing through the vaporizer. With a VOC, vapour concentration in the circle falls below that dialled up as the fresh gas flow is diluted by the exhaled gases; it therefore takes a long time to adjust the vapour concentration at low flows and rapid adjustments should be achieved by temporarily increasing the flow rates. It is important to monitor the vapour concentrations delivered to the patient if low flows (below 2 l/min) are used. Very low flows (below 1 l/min) are easily possible but care must be taken to monitor both oxygen and vapour concentrations delivered to the patient. The minimum flow in a system at equilibrium with no leaks is delivery of the amount of oxygen consumed by the patient (approximately 200 ml/min); in practice a minimum flow rate of 500 ml/min is usually set.

70. **Suitable methods for disinfection of a laryngoscope blade include:**
    A. soaking in 2% activated glutaraldehyde solution for 20 min.
    B. boiling for 5 min.
    C. pasteurization.
    D. soaking in 0.05% chlorhexidine solution for 30 min.
    E. soaking in a water bath at 70°C for 5 min.

71. **Pulse oximeter readings are inaccurate in the presence of the following conditions.**
    A. mild anaemia.
    B. methaemoglobinaemia.
    C. carboxyhaemoglobinaemia.
    D. sickle cell anaemia.
    E. hyperbilirubinaemia.

70. ABCD

Cleaning of anaesthetic apparatus can involve the following processes:

decontamination: physical removal of infected matter and debris

disinfection: killing all infective organisms apart from the most resistant spores

sterilization: killing of all organisms including spores.

Physical methods

Heating: dry or moist

Filtration, e.g. glass sinter

Radiation, e.g. γ (cobalt 60) irradiation for 2 days

Ethylene oxide gas

Autoclaving

Pasteurization is one of the easiest ways to disinfect equipment and consists of heating to a temperature of 70°C for 20 min or 80°C for 10 min. Boiling in water for 5 min also disinfects

Chemical methods

Isopropyl alcohol

Chlorhexidine solution (0.05%) for 30 min

Chloroxylenol

2% Glutaraldehyde

Hypochlorite solutions

---

71. BCE

There are a number of potential sources of error in pulse oximeter readings: the presence of abnormal haemoglobins such as methaemoglobin and carboxyhaemoglobin or in neonates high levels of fetal haemoglobins; dyes or pigments such as methylene blue or nail varnish; motion or vibration may cause an artefact; a powerful ambient light source can flood the photodiode; pulsation of the venous bed (i.e. tricuspid incompetence). Anaemia and sickle cell anaemia do not affect the readings, whilst hyperbilirubinaemia reads falsely low, carboxyhaemoglobinaemia consistently reads at 100% and methaemoglobinaemia consistently reads at 85%.

72. **The following are minimum monitoring requirements as recommended by the Association of Anaesthetists of Great Britain and Ireland:**
    A. continuous monitoring of ventilation.
    B. the presence of an anaesthetist from induction to recovery.
    C. capnography must be available for every case.
    D. monitoring of the oxygen concentration at the common gas outlet is essential.
    E. the monitoring recommendations only apply to patients undergoing general anaesthesia.

73. **Pulse oximeters:**
    A. give falsely high readings in the presence of myoglobin.
    B. are a useful monitor of oxygenation and ventilation in recovery.
    C. work on the principle of absorption spectrophotometry.
    D. work on the principle that oxygenated haemoglobin absorbs light of wavelength 910 nm.
    E. utilise the Lambert–Beer law.

72. ABCD
Recommendations for the standards of monitoring during anaesthesia were published by the Association of Anaesthetists of Great Britain and Ireland and are intended to apply to patients being administered general, regional or local anaesthesia or undergoing sedation where there is a risk of unconsciousness developing.

Association of Anaesthetists of Great Britain and Ireland (1994) *Recommendations for Standards of Monitoring during Anaesthesia and Recovery*, revised edn. The Association of Anaesthetists of Great Britain and Ireland, London.

73. CDE
Pulse oximeters work on the principle of absorption spectrophotometry. They consist of a light-emitting diode that alternately transmits red and infra red light through an extremity (usually the finger). A photodetector then reads the incident light and a ratio is determined between the different absorption of the two wavelengths of light. Only the light that is constantly varying (representing the arterial component) is used by the microprocessor in the calculations. Reduced and oxygenated haemoglobin absorb different amounts of light at different wavelengths (maximally at 660 and 910 nm respectively), except at the isobestic point (803 nm) where the absorption is identical. Pulse oximeters are calibrated for adult haemoglobin. The pulse oximeter measures the pulsatile differences between oxyhaemoglobin and deoxyhaemoglobin and, using the Lambert–Beer law works out the percentage saturation. The Lambert–Beer law states that two substances of equal thickness will absorb radiation equally and that absorption of radiation by a solution is proportional to its concentration. It is important to remember that pulse oximeters do not give a measure of the adequacy of *ventilation* especially if supplemental oxygen is being given.

74. **Visual or tactile assessment of the degree of neuromuscular blockade can be made by the following:**
    A. double burst stimulation.
    B. a train-of-four stimulus at 50 Hz.
    C. a tetanic train of 5 Hz for 5 s.
    D. a post-tetanic twitch at 1 Hz.
    E. ability to maintain arterial oxygen saturation above 90%.

75. **The following are true regarding capnographs:**
    A. they usually work on the principle of infrared absorption.
    B. sidestream analysers have a longer response time than mainstream analysers.
    C. they must be calibrated regularly.
    D. they may give a transient carbon dioxide waveform during accidental oesophageal intubation.
    E. they will give a rapid indication of accidental endo-bronchial intubation.

74. AD

Assessment of neuromuscular blockade may involve the following:

supramaximal stimulation of the nerve terminals must be produced by supplying an adequate current (50 mA) of sufficient duration (0.2–1.0 ms);

a train of single shocks given at a rate of one every 3 s;

a tetanic burst at 50 Hz for 5 s followed by a post-tetanic twitch rate of 1/s (1 Hz);

a train-of-four stimulus at 0.5-s intervals (2 Hz); it may be repeated every 10 s without significant loss of accuracy:

two short lasting 50 Hz tetanic stimuli (3 impulses in each stimulus) separated by 0.75 seconds (double burst stimulation).

75. ABCD

Capnographs work on the principle of infrared absorption spectroscopy. They need to be calibrated regularly using a gas containing a known concentration of carbon dioxide according to the manufacturer's instructions; most modern machines carry out a regular automatic zero calibration. There are two main types of capnographs.

Sidestream analysers have the advantage of being lightweight and the sampling is done close to the trachea. Disadvantages include condensation of vapour along the sampling line, a longer response time and removal of between 50 and 150 ml/min of gas flow.

Mainstream analysers have the advantage that the gas never leaves the breathing circuit and there is a minimal response time. The main disadvantage is that of a cumbersome piece of equipment at the patient end of the breathing system.

Although the gold standard for confirming tracheal intubation is the presence of carbon dioxide in the expired gas, this may rarely occur for the first few breaths when oesophageal intubation has occurred, especially if carbonated drinks have recently been consumed. Endobronchial intubation will not be detected by capnography.

O'Flaherty, D. (1994) *Capnography.* British Medical Journal Publishing, London.

76. **The application of cricoid pressure in a rapid sequence induction:**
   A. was first described by Magill.
   B. may make tracheal intubation more difficult.
   C. should be applied with a force of approximately 44 N.
   D. should be maintained if the patient starts actively vomiting.
   E. should be fully applied before induction of anaesthesia.

77. **Methaemoglobinaemia:**
   A. occurs when the ferrous form of iron in haemoglobin is oxidized to the ferric form.
   B. causes a cherry red colour in the fingertips.
   C. causes a shift to the right in the oxygen–haemoglobin dissociation curve.
   D. may be caused by inhalation of nitric oxide.
   E. is treated with *n*-acetylcysteine.

76. BC

Prevention of aspiration of stomach contents following regurgitation by the application of cricoid pressure was first described by Sellick, hence the alternative name of Sellick's manoeuvre. When correctly applied, a force of 44 N is required to prevent regurgitation; this force, however, is too great for the awake patient to tolerate, so it should be applied immediately after induction of anaesthesia or gradually during induction. If active vomiting occurs, cricoid pressure should be released because of the risk of oesophageal rupture.

77. AD

Methaemoglobinaemia occurs in the following situations:

congenital: an autosomal recessive condition resulting in absence of the enzyme reduced nicotinamide adenine dinucleotide (NADH) diaphorase

acquired: poisoning with amyl nitrate, prilocaine, sulphonamides and phenacetin, and treatment with nitric oxide.

Symptoms occur when 20% of the haemoglobin becomes methaemoglobin and the patient becomes cyanosed; in extreme conditions haemolysis and disseminated intravascular coagulopathy occur. There is a shift to the left in the oxygen–haemoglobin dissociation curve and pulse oximeter readings are lower than the actual level (i.e. under-read). Treatment is with vitamin C for the congenital condition and methylene blue (1 mg/kg i.v.) for drug poisoning.

78. **The following factors can be shown to have an association with difficult orotracheal intubation by conventional laryngoscopy:**
    A. the patient is diabetic and over 40 years of age.
    B. the thyromental distance is less than 6.5 cm.
    C. the patient suffers from Marfan's syndrome.
    D. there is bilateral recurrent laryngeal nerve palsy.
    E. Mallampati class 1.

79. **The following morbidity is paired correctly with patient position during surgery:**
    A. common peroneal nerve damage and lithotomy.
    B. inferior vena caval compression and nephrectomy position.
    C. 30% reduction in cardiac output with a Trendelenburg tilt.
    D. facial oedema and the prone position.
    E. tongue oedema and the sitting position.

80. **The following may result from impaired humidification of inspired gases in a long-term intubated patient:**
    A. changes in tracheal cytology.
    B. increase in pulmonary compliance.
    C. decreased functional residual capacity.
    D. atelectasis.
    E. increased alveolar–arterial pulmonary shunting.

78.   **ABC**

Both diabetes (especially if cheirarthropathy is present) and age over 40 years are separately associated with difficult intubation. The thyromental distance (as described by Patil) should be measured in full neck extension; it can be conveniently measured in fingerbreadths, and in one study the minimum distance was three fingerbreadths (or 6.5 cm), less than this being associated with difficulty with intubation. Marfan's syndrome is the combination of lax ligaments, high arched palate and aortic root disease. With bilateral recurrent laryngeal nerve palsies, the cords should adopt the cadaveric mid-position and there is no difficulty in passing a tracheal tube between them. Mallampati class 3 is associated with difficult intubation and is characterized by seeing only the tongue pressed against the palate on full mouth opening. In class 1 a full view is obtained of the posterior pharyngeal wall and fauces.

79.   **BDE**

The common peroneal nerve crosses the neck of the fibula on the lateral side of the calf. In the lithotomy position, the legs should be placed outside the poles so that the common peroneal nerves are not affected. Incidentally, the commonest palsy occurring during anaesthesia is of the ulnar nerve, and this has been reported several times more commonly in men than in women. The Trendelenburg position was associated with brachial plexus lesions when shoulder pads were used to prevent the patient sliding off the table in a steep head down tilt.

80.   **ACDE**

The following are all recognized hazards of impaired humidification of inspired gases:

>   increased desquamation of cells, dessication of mucosa, changes in tracheal cytology with squamous metaplasia
>   increase in sputum viscosity and mucous airway plugs
>   loss of ciliary function
>   increased airway resistance and decreased pulmonary compliance
>   atelectasis and decreased functional residual capacity
>   loss of surfactant
>   increased alveolar–arterial shunting
>   hypothermia.

81. **The following features are desirable in a patient-controlled analgesia (PCA) delivery system:**
    A. small size.
    B. simplicity of use.
    C. facility for the patient to adjust the delivered dose.
    D. preset dose prescription regimens.
    E. free flow.

82. **When considering anaesthesia at high altitude (above 10 000 feet):**
    A. nitrous oxide is an effective analgesic.
    B. the partial pressure of vapours delivered by a plenum vaporizer are reduced significantly.
    C. the density of gases decreases.
    D. a minimum inspired oxygen concentration of 40% is recommended.
    E. fixed performance oxygen masks will deliver less than the indicated oxygen concentration.

83. **The following items of anaesthetic equipment need to be recalibrated when used at high altitude (above 10 000 feet):**
    A. paramagnetic oxygen analysers.
    B. fuel cell oxygen analysers.
    C. capnographs.
    D. pulse oximeters.
    E. flowmeters.

81. **AB**
A PCA delivery system should have the following features:

safety
simplicity
small size and easy portability
security against tampering
ability to record patient demands and drug usage
prevention of free flow
versatility for different administration modes and drug
    prescriptions
alarms to detect malfunction.

82. **CD**

83. **ABCE**
At altitude the reduction in atmospheric pressure results in a proportional reduction in the partial pressures of inspired gases. It is therefore recommended that the inspired oxygen concentration is increased to 40% when administering a gas mixture above 5000 feet. Nitrous oxide is a poor analgesic at moderate altitude and its effect is insignificant at altitudes above 10 000 feet. The density of a gas decreases with altitude, whereas the viscosity remains unchanged. The fixed-orifice Venturi mask will therefore deliver a higher concentration of oxygen than at sea level, provided the flowmeter used is properly calibrated. The saturated vapour pressure of a volatile anaesthetic agent does not depend on temperature and as atmospheric pressure decreases the same mass of volatile agent is vaporized in less dense carrier gas; therefore the actual concentration of vapour delivered increases but the partial pressure (and its clinical effect) remains constant. All gas analysers that respond to the number of molecules of a gas that are present will need to be recalibrated at altitude, or under-reading will occur.

84. **The following agents are correctly paired with their cylinder colours:**

		Body	Shoulder
A.	oxygen	black	white
B.	carbon dioxide	grey	white
C.	nitrous oxide	blue	white
D.	air	black	grey/white
E.	entonox	blue	blue

85. **The following are true with regard to defibrillator machines:**
    A. they were first used in clinical practice in the early 1960s.
    B. the impedance of a patient is typically approximately 5 ohms.
    C. synchronized shock is delivered at the start of the R wave of the QRS complex.
    D. impedance is increased if no electrode pads are used.
    E. the most effective position for the electrode pads is over the sternum and left lateral chest wall.

86. **The following may lead to hypercarbia during controlled ventilation:**
    A. low fresh gas flow in a circle system.
    B. Bain circuit tubing longer than 3 m.
    C. decreased apparatus deadspace.
    D. lack of a unidirectional valve in a circle system.
    E. increasing the expiratory time on a Penlon Nuffield 200 ventilator.

84. A

	Body	Shoulder
oxygen	black	white
carbon dioxide	grey	grey
nitrous oxide	blue	blue
air	grey	white/black quarters
entonox	blue	white/blue quarters

85. D

Defibrillation was first introduced into clinical practice in 1947 when electrodes were applied directly to the heart. Closed chest defibrillation with alternating current (AC) was introduced in 1956. A defibrillator delivers direct current rather than AC, which cannot synchronize with the electrocardiogram (ECG). Charge is stored in a capacitor, and energy available is equal to half the charge (160 mC (milliCoulombs)) multiplied by the voltage (5000 V), producing 400 J. Synchronized shock delivers the energy 20 ms after the start of the R wave of the ECG. The jelly placed on the electrode pads reduces the impedance to the heart (normally approximately 50 ohms), and the most effective positions for the pads are on the front and back of the chest wall so that energy is delivered across the heart; however, for practical reasons the sternum and lateral chest wall are sufficient in most cases.

86. DE

Hypercarbia will not occur in a circle system if the unidirectional valves are working properly, although great care must be taken to ensure that the correct gas mixture and concentration of volatile anaesthetic agent are reaching the patient at low gas flows. The Bain breathing system has no limitation in its effective length: circuits 10 m in length are used in special situations with no changes in the physical properties. Increased apparatus deadspace may lead to hypercarbia, especially in infants and neonates. The Penlon Nuffield 200 ventilator produces a controlled rebreathing situation; for the carbon dioxide level to increase, either the fresh gas flow to the circuit must be reduced or the respiratory rate reduced.

87. **When considering conditions of increased barometric pressure under water:**
    A. pressure increases by 1 atmosphere for each 33 m of descent.
    B. nitrogen narcosis occurs at pressures of 3 atmospheres.
    C. grand mal seizures occur if 100% oxygen is breathed at 3 atmospheres' pressure.
    D. decompression sickness is due to gas bubble formation in blood and tissues.
    E. solubility of gases decreases with increasing depth under water.

88. **When considering anaesthesia within a magnetic resonance imaging (MRI) suite:**
    A. waveguides are required for all cables and wires.
    B. ECG complexes are always distorted.
    C. electromagnetic interference affects oscillotonometric blood pressure measurement.
    D. capnography is of little use because of electromagnetic interference.
    E. temperature monitoring is recommended because of the risks of hypothermia.

89. **The following marks are found on anaesthetic gas cylinders:**
    A. date of pressure testing.
    B. name of contents.
    C. chemical formula of contents.
    D. weight of empty cylinder.
    E. volume of cylinder contents.

90. **The desflurance TEC Mk 6 vaporizer:**
    A. heats desflurane to a temperature of 23.5°C.
    B. has a dial calibrated from 0 to 10%.
    C. can be used inside a magnetic resonance imaging (MRI) room.
    D. has a capacity of approximately 450 ml.
    E. has fresh gas flow entering the vaporization chamber.

87. CD

Barometric pressure under water increases by 1 atmosphere for every 10 m (or 33 feet) of descent. Nitrogen starts to exert a pharmacological effect at pressures of around 5 atmospheres and narcosis is seen at pressures exceeding 8–10 atmospheres. Air may be breathed safely at pressures of 3 atmospheres for prolonged periods of time with no harmful effects; however, when 100% oxygen is breathed at 3 atmospheres' pressure, oxygen toxicity, including grand mal seizures, occurs rapidly. The solubility of gases increases with increasing pressure and if decompression occurs rapidly gas bubbles may form in blood and tissues, leading to decompression sickness.

88. AB

Capnography is a very useful monitor of ventilation in the MRI suite, although there may be a prolonged time lag owing to the length of the tubing. Temperature should be monitored because radiofrequency raises body temperature.

89. ACD

Modern anaesthetic gas and vapour cylinders are made of molybdenum steel, are colour coded and have the following markings:

> tare weight (weight of empty cylinder)
> chemical formula of the contents
> test pressure
> date of pressure testing
> name of the owner
> serial number of the cylinder.

90. D

Desflurance boils at 23.5°C and a special vaporizer (TEC Mk 6) was developed to deliver desflurane vapour; an electrically heated chamber with a capacity of 450 ml heats desflurane to a temperature of 39°C and pressure of 1550 mmHg. None of the fresh gas flow enters the vaporizer, the desflurane being released into the fresh gas flow according to a dialled up concentration from 0 to 18%. The vaporizer is ferromagnetic and cannot be used inside an MRI scanner.

Paper 2

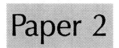

1. **Remifentanil:**
   A. is a pure μ-opioid receptor agonist.
   B. is metabolized by plasma cholinesterase.
   C. has clinically active metabolites.
   D. is equipotent with alfentanil.
   E. does not cause nausea and vomiting.

2. **Digoxin:**
   A. is a negative inotropic agent.
   B. increases the excitability of the heart.
   C. causes an increase in intracellular calcium in cardiac muscle.
   D. may cause gynaecomastia.
   E. requires increased dosage in the elderly.

1. **A**

   Remifentanil is a new pure μ-opioid receptor agonist which is a fentanyl derivative (and has similar pharmacodynamic proper-ties to fentanyl) and contains an ester linkage. It has a similar speed of onset as alfentanil but is 15–30 times more potent, has a volume of distribution of 25–40 l, and is 70% plasma protein bound. Remifentanil is rapidly broken down by non-specific esterases (its terminal half life is 10–21 min) to metabolites which have approximately 0.2% of the activity of remifentanil. It has a clearance of 4.2–5 l/min and this remains constant regardless of age, sex, weight and renal or hepatic dysfunction, and the context-sensitive half-time (the time for the effect site concentration to fall by 50% after terminating an infusion designed to maintain a constant plasma concentration) is approximately 3.6 min after a 3-hour infusion. Remifentanil is a poor substrate for plasma cholinesterase and is therefore unaffected by cholinesterase deficiency. At present remifentanil is formulated in glycine and is therefore unsuitable for intrathecal or epidural use. Another potential problem is that significant pain may be experienced by the patient shortly after discontinuation of remifentanil, and other forms of analgesia will be required in the postoperative period.

2. **BCD**

   Digoxin is a cardiac glycoside that enhances myocardial contraction and decreases conduction at the atrioventricular node. The mechanism of action is by inhibition of the enzyme Na^+-K^+ ATPase, leading to a rise in intracellular sodium and calcium. The main clinical indications are in the control of atrial tachyarrhythmias and cardiac failure. It has a low therapeutic index and the incidence of toxicity is worsened by hypokalaemia. Digoxin is excreted by the kidney and reduced doses are required in the elderly. It may cause bradyarrhythmias including complete heart block, as well as a wide range of ventricular arrhythmias from isolated ectopics to ventricular tachycardia and fibrillation. Other side-effects include anorexia, nausea and vomiting, lethargy and disorientation, neuralgic pains, blurred vision and gynaecomastia. Treatment of toxicity is by cessation of oral therapy, correction of electrolyte abnormalities and appropriate treatment of any resulting arrhythmias. Measures may be taken to decrease absorption of digoxin from the gastrointestinal tract and in severe cases fragmented digoxin antibodies may be given.

3. **Nitric oxide (NO):**
   A. is a gas.
   B. has a strong affinity for haemoglobin.
   C. must be administered in a concentration of at least 50 parts per million (ppm) for clinical effect.
   D. dilates pulmonary blood vessels.
   E. is usually stored in cylinders mixed with nitrogen.

4. **The use of a non-specific β-adrenergic blocker in the treatment of hypertension:**
   A. may cause exacerbation of asthma.
   B. often produces postural hypotension.
   C. is contraindicated in patients with high renin levels.
   D. may cause cardiac failure in susceptible patients.
   E. should be avoided if Raynaud's phenomenon is present.

3. **ABDE**

NO is a gas that is widely distributed in the body. It has important regulatory roles in the circulatory system, as well as in the nervous and immune systems. Previously known as endothelial-derived relaxing factor (EDRF), NO is synthesized from one of the terminal nitrogen atoms of L-arginine in a stereospecific process catalysed by the enzyme nitric oxide synthetase (NOS). Several isoforms of NOS exist and some are inducible. After production in the vascular endothelial cell NO diffuses to the smooth muscle cell where it activates guanylate cyclase leading to an increase in cyclic guanosine monophosphate (cGMP) and thence to muscle relaxation and vasodilatation. Disorders of NO metabolism underly many disease states including endotoxic shock, in which prolonged production of NO may be induced by cytokines. NO is administered by inhalation in carefully controlled concentrations in the range of 5–20 ppm. Its duration of action is a few seconds only. In tissues NO degrades to nitrates and nitrites with little biological action, and in blood it combines with haemoglobin. The resulting nitrosyl-haemoglobin is oxidized to methaemoglobin. Although it is a non-specific vasodilator, its brief duration of action and administration via inhalation result in pronounced pulmonary, rather than systemic, vasodilatation. Nitrogen dioxide is a noxious agent and is a time-related product of the reaction between NO and oxygen and may be a contaminant of preparations of NO.

4. **ADE**

The β-adrenergic blockers are specifically contraindicated in second- and third-degree heart block, asthma and prolonged fasting. They should be used with care in patients with poor cardiac reserve, peripheral vascular disease and in diabetic patients. A rebound phenomenon also occurs if they are discontinued abruptly. Side-effects include depression, hallucinations and nightmares, insomnia, lethargy and gastrointestinal upset. Postural hypotension is a common side-effect of the α-blocking agents resulting from peripheral vasodilatation.

5. **The following statements about osmotic diuretics are correct:**
   A. they are only effective if they are completely reabsorbed in the renal tubule.
   B. they reduce intracranial pressure primarily by inducing a diuresis.
   C. intravenous sucrose can reduce intracranial pressure.
   D. pulmonary oedema may result from their use if renal function is impaired.
   E. urea can produce a useful diuresis in patients with renal failure.

5. **CD**

Osmotic diuretics such as mannitol (a polyhydric alcohol with a molecular weight of 180), urea or sucrose act because they are filtered across the glomerulus but are not reabsorbed by the renal tubules and hence are excreted with an isosmotic equivalent volume of water. These agents induce diuresis despite the action of antidiuretic hormone (ADH) and the most marked loss is that of water rather than salt. The principal mode of action in reducing cerebral oedema is by an osmotic effect, causing shrinkage of brain cells because water is drawn into the intravascular space. In addition there is evidence that mannitol may act as a free radical scavenger and may be of use in preventing reperfusion damage following head injury. Osmotic diuretics cause an increase in renal plasma flow and increased intraluminal pressure and this helps prevent the development of acute renal failure in predisposing conditions such as oliguria associated with major surgery or trauma. In established renal failure, the water drawn into the intravascular space cannot be eliminated and this may lead to hypervolaemic hyponatraemia or to the development of pulmonary oedema. Urea is as effective as mannitol in patients with normal renal function but has other side-effects, such as cardiac arrhythmias, haemolysis and can cause an increase in bleeding tendency.

6. **The following drugs inhibit reuptake of released noradrenaline by sympathetic nerve terminals:**
   A. pancuronium.
   B. guanethidine.
   C. reserpine.
   D. bretylium.
   E. clonidine.

7. **The following drugs may cause pulmonary oedema:**
   A. adrenaline.
   B. atropine.
   C. opioids.
   D. nifedipine.
   E. cyclophosphamide.

6. **ABC**

The action of noradrenaline at sympathetic nerve terminals is terminated in two ways: firstly by the uptake of noradrenaline by the presynaptic membrane (uptake 1) where it is recycled back into the vesicular stores; and secondly by uptake into the postsynaptic membrane (uptake 2) where it is broken down by monoamine oxidase (MAO) and catechol-*O*-methyltransferase (COMT). Drugs that block uptake therefore act as indirect sympathomimetics. These include ephedrine, amphetamine, tyramine and cocaine. Reserpine in low concentration is also a noradrenergic reuptake blocker but at higher concentrations prevents storage of noradrenaline by damaging the vesicle membrane so depleting transmitter stores. Pancuronium is a non-depolarizing neuromuscular blocking agent that also has some sympathomimetic activity caused by blockade of noradrenaline reuptake. It also acts as a muscarinic receptor blocker. Clonidine is a centrally acting α_2 agonist that causes a reduction in transmitter release. Bretylium has adrenergic neurone-blocking properties caused by its accumulation in the sympathetic ganglia with a subsequent decrease in noradrenaline release. It may however have an initial sympathomimetic effect caused by transient discharge of noradrenaline. Guanethidine is a sympatholytic agent and works by inhibition of reuptake, leading to depleted vesicles.

7. **ACE**

Pulmonary oedema may occur if pulmonary capillary pressure is high, pulmonary capillary permeability is increased or oncotic pressure is reduced. Any sympathomimetic capable of producing intense vasoconstriction can cause pulmonary oedema by increasing lung capillary pressure. Although diamorphine is commonly used to treat cardiogenic pulmonary oedema, opioid poisoning causes an increase in vascular permeability that can result in pulmonary oedema (either bilateral or unilateral). When pulmonary oedema accompanies an opioid overdose, it is difficult to separate a drug effect from possible aspiration pneumonitis or hypoxia-induced acute lung injury. Cyclophosphamide in high doses may cause cardiotoxicity and this may lead to intractable heart failure and pulmonary oedema.

8. **Aprotinin:**
   A. is an antifibrinolytic.
   B. is associated with an increased risk of thrombosis if given to normal patients.
   C. is synthetic.
   D. reduces blood loss following open heart surgery.
   E. helps protect platelet function.

9. **If applied topically to the cornea:**
   A. cocaine will result in loss of the corneal reflex.
   B. cocaine will dilate the pupil.
   C. physostigmine will constrict the pupil.
   D. physostigmine will impair accommodation for near vision.
   E. amethocaine will dilate the pupil.

8   ADE

Aprotinin is a polypeptide protease inhibitor derived from bovine lung tissue and marketed under the trade name Trasylol. It is an inhibitor of proteolytic enzymes including human trypsin, plasmin, and both tissue and plasma kallikrein. It acts as an inhibitor of fibrinolysis, has been used in the treatment of pancreatitis, maintains platelet adhesiveness and attenuates the intrinsic clotting pathway. It has been shown to reduce blood loss in a variety of surgical procedures including open heart surgery. The recommended dosage in open heart surgery is a loading dose of 2 million KIU (kallikrein inhibitory units) prior to sternotomy followed by 0.5 million KIU/hour until the end of surgery. The principal serious side-effects are anaphylactoid hypersensitivity reactions and renal impairment.

9.   ABC

Pupillary dilatation is under the control of the iris sphincter muscle, which is constricted by its parasympathetic nerve supply and dilated by its sympathetic nerve supply. Accommodation for near vision is regulated by the ciliary muscle, which is under parasympathetic control; therefore muscarinic antagonists paralyse the muscle and prevent accommodation for near vision, whilst muscarinic agonists cause ciliary muscle constitution and loss of far vision. Cocaine has both local anaesthetic and sympathomimetic properties and physostigmine is an anticholinesterase (i.e. a cholinergic agonist).

10. **The following may prolong the Q–T interval on the ECG:**
    A. amiodarone.
    B. disopyramide.
    C. terfenadine.
    D. chlorpromazine.
    E. hypocalcaemia.

10. ABCDE

The Q–T interval on the ECG is measured from the beginning of the QRS complex to the end of the T wave. The normal Q–T interval varies with heart rate, but the rate-corrected Q–T duration (QT$_c$) is described by Bazetts formula as the Q–T interval divided by the square root of the R–R interval and has an upper limit of 440 ms or approximately 50% of the R–R interval. A Q–T interval of greater than 550 ms predisposes to ventricular arrhythmias. Causes of a prolonged Q–T interval are numerous and are shown in the table.

Medical causes

Ischaemic heart disease, mitral valve prolapse

Rheumatic carditis, pulmonary embolus

Raised intracranial pressure, familial syndromes, e.g. Romano–Ward syndrome

Metabolic causes

Hypothyroidism, hypothermia, hypocalcaemia

Drug causes

Quinidine, disopyramide, amiodarone, sotalol

Tricyclic antidepressants

Antipsychotics such as phenothiazines

Terfenadine

Committee on Safety of Medicines and Medicines Control Agency (1996) Drug induced prolongation of the QT interval. *Current Problems in Pharmacovigilance* **22**, 2.

Thomas, S.H.L. (1997) Drugs and the QT interval. *Adverse Drug Reactions Bulletin* **182**, 691–694.

11. **Desflurane:**
    A. is a fluorinated methyl ether.
    B. has a minimum alveolar concentration (MAC) value of 2%.
    C. has a blood:gas solubility of 0.42.
    D. is flammable in a concentration of 6%.
    E. should not be used with soda lime.

12. **The barrier pressure between the lower oesophagus and the stomach is increased by:**
    A. neostigmine.
    B. atropine.
    C. suxamethonium.
    D. thiopentone.
    E. antacids.

11. AC

Desflurane is a fluorinated methyl ether (formula $CF_3CFHOCF_2H$, molecular weight 168) with a very low blood: gas solubility of 0.42 and an MAC value of 6%. It has a high saturated vapour pressure (664 mmHg) due to its low boiling point (23.5°C), which makes it unsuitable for use in traditional vaporizers. These problems have been overcome by the use of an electronic vaporizer that heats the desflurane, converting it into a vapour. The agent is ideally suited to low flow systems since it does not react with soda lime and because its low solubility allows rapid induction of anaesthesia. Desflurane has similar effects to isoflurane on the cardiovascular system: it decreases systemic vascular resistance, cardiac output and mean arterial pressure and increases heart rate, but it does not appear to cause the 'coronary steal' thought to occur with isoflurane. (See figure in Paper 1, question 14.)

12. ACE

The lower oesophageal sphincter (LOS) is an area of higher resting intraluminal pressure in the region of the stomach cardia that cannot be defined anatomically but which prevents reflux of gastric contents into the oesophagus. It is not the actual LOS tone that is important but the difference between LOS and intragastric pressure – the barrier pressure – which prevents reflux. Normally, a cholinergic reflex loop acts to increase LOS tone in the presence of raised intragastric or intra-abdominal pressure. Certain drugs such as suxamethonium cause an increase in intragastric pressure but also cause a greater increase in LOS pressure, which results in an overall increase in the barrier pressure.

Drugs which increase barrier pressure	Drugs which lower barrier pressure
Prochlorperazine, cisapride, domperidone, cyclizine	Anticholinergics
Anticholinesterases (neostigmine)	Thiopentone, volatile anaesthetic agents
α-Adrenergic agonists	Tricyclic antidepressants
Suxamethonium	Ganglion blockers
Antacids (via an increase in pH)	Ethanol

13. **When a blood transfusion reaction is suspected:**
    A. the infusion rate should be reduced and the label checked.
    B. the only signs during surgery under general anaesthesia may be hypotension and generalized wound ooze.
    C. the usual cause of a haemolytic reaction is clerical error.
    D. an IgG response is the usual immunological response to incompatible transfusion.
    E. blood samples should be taken from the patient for future analysis.

13. BCE

Approximately 2% of blood transfusions are followed by some form of reaction, about 75% of these being febrile reactions due to HLA antigens. Haemolytic reactions involving ABO incompatibility are much rarer, may be fatal and are often (75%) due to clerical error. Other transfusion reactions may be mediated by IgA or graft vs host in immunocompromised patients. During anaesthesia the only signs of a major haemolytic reaction may be tachycardia, hypotension and generalized wound ooze; other signs are oliguria and haemoglobinuria. If a transfusion reaction is suspected the transfusion should be stopped immediately and a check made for any clerical errors. The urine output should be monitored hourly and oliguria treated initially by maintenance of normovolaemia and frusemide. The plasma potassium should be measured frequently and hyperkalaemia treated initially with dextrose and insulin. Blood samples should be taken from the patient and returned to the transfusion department together with the remaining donor blood. A raised urinary haemoglobin is indicative of haemolysis. Mild pyrexial transfusion reactions may be prevented by a white cell filter, and urticaria by pretreatment with chlorpheniramine.

14. **The following cause a reduction in pseudocholinesterase activity:**
    A. pregnancy.
    B. obesity.
    C. hypothyroidism.
    D. alcohol.
    E. pancuronium.

14. ACE

Cholinesterases are enzymes that hydrolyse acetylcholine and other choline esters at a more rapid rate than non-choline esters. There are two types of cholinesterase: red cell, also known as true or specific, cholinesterase is found in human erythrocytes and nervous tissue and is highly specific for acetylcholine; pseudo or non-specific cholinesterase is found in plasma and hydrolyses a wider range of choline esters. Reduction in pseudocholinesterase activity occurs in the conditions shown in the table.

Physiological variation	Newborn, pregnancy
Inherited	Suxamethonium apnoea
Medical conditions	Liver disease, malignancy, malnutrition, severe heart failure, end-stage renal failure, burns, hypothyroidism
Drugs	Oral contraceptive pill, cyclophosphamide, ecothiopate (usually given as eyedrops), neostigmine and the other reversible cholinesterase inhibitors, pancuronium, metoclopramide
Others	Organophosphate and carbamate pesticides, plasmapheresis, cardiopulmonary bypass

Increased activity has been demonstrated in hyperthyroidism, obesity, nephrotic syndrome, psoriasis, alcoholics, non-specific mental illness and mental retardation.

Davis, L., Britten, J.J., Morgan, M. (1997) Cholinesterase: its significance in clinical practice. *Anaesthesia* **52**, 244–60.

15. **Ketamine:**
    A. increases cerebral blood flow.
    B. is an *N*-methyl-*D*-aspartate (NMDA) receptor agonist.
    C. causes a reduction in airway secretions.
    D. is a poor analgesic.
    E. causes premature labour contractions.

16. **Low molecular weight heparins:**
    A. contain unfractionated heparins.
    B. are usually given twice daily.
    C. should be monitored during use by the activated partial thromboplastin time (APTT).
    D. should be discontinued at least 6 hours before major surgery.
    E. may cause thrombocytopenia if given for more than 1 week.

15. A

Ketamine is a phencyclidine derivative that produces dissociative anaesthesia. It is an organic base with a pK_a of 7.5. The usual dose for induction of anaesthesia is 1–2 mg/kg i.v. or 5–10 mg/kg i.m. It undergoes redistribution with a half-life of 10 min and is metabolized in the liver with an elimination half-life of 3 hours. It is a powerful analgesic in subanaesthetic concentrations and is a non-competitive antagonist at NMDA receptors (usually mediated by L-glutamate). Ketamine maintains cardiovascular stability and, in contrast to other anaesthetic induction agents, causes an increase in blood pressure that is associated with a tachycardia. It causes minimal respiratory depression when used alone and is a powerful bronchodilator but does, however, cause copious secretions and pretreatment with a drying agent is advisable. It causes an increase in cerebral blood flow and cerebral oxygen consumption which may result in an increase in intracranial pressure. Recovery from anaesthesia is complicated by vivid emergence phenomena and hallucinations, which can be reduced by recovery in a dark, calm environment and by the administration of benzodiazepines. Ketamine does not cause premature labour but does enhance the tone and pressure of established uterine contractions and should be avoided in situations where enhanced uterine activity may be harmful, e.g. umbilical cord prolapse or placental abruption. The commercial preparation is racemic and consists of *S* and *R* enantiomers. The *S* (+) form is more potent and produces less emergence phenomena.

16. E

Low molecular weight heparins are fractionated heparins with a long half-life. The bioavailability following subcutaneous administration is 90%, with a peak onset of action of 4–6 hours. They are given once daily in a dose of 5000 iu subcutaneously. It is not necessary to monitor the APTT as this is not affected by the heparin. It can safely be given up to 1–2 hours preoperatively for deep vein thrombosis prophylaxis, but if given for more than 1 week the platelet count can decrease and should be monitored.

17. **In clinical dosage, captopril:**
    A. may cause hyperkalaemia.
    B. may cause a dry cough.
    C. should be given with food.
    D. is given orally once daily.
    E. causes an increased level of angiotensin I.

18. **Gelofusine:**
    A. is derived from human plasma.
    B. contains molecules with an average molecular weight of 30 000.
    C. contains calcium.
    D. contains sodium chloride.
    E. may cause hypersensitivity reactions.

17. ABE

Captopril is an angiotensin-converting enzyme (ACE) inhibitor usually administered orally 8-hourly. It is not a prodrug, unlike many other ACE inhibitors. It should be taken 1 hour before meals because food reduces bioavailability by 25%. Side-effects include hypotension, elevation of serum creatinine, protein-uria, hyperkalaemia, rash, troublesome cough (in up to 15% of patients), angioedema, neutropenia and taste disorders. Potentiation of the effects of lithium have been reported. The drug may be used in patients suffering from hypertension or left ventricular dysfunction. It is probable that the use of ACE inhibitors for heart failure leads to an improved survival when compared with placebo. Whilst acute renal insufficiency can occur in patients with renal artery stenosis or overtreated with diuretics, it appears to retard the loss of kidney function in diabetic nephropathy. ACE inhibitors impair regulation of the normal renin–angiotensin axis but the increased levels of angiotensin I do not appear to produce an adverse effect.

18. BDE

Gelofusine is a gelatine-based compound containing molecules with an average molecular weight of 30 000. It is derived by hydrolysis and succinylation of collagen from bovine hooves. It contains sodium chloride 154 mmol/l and has an osmolarity of 279 mosmol/l but, unlike Haemaccel, does not contain calcium. Gelofusine can cause hypersensitivity reactions and the reported frequency of severe reactions is from 1:6000 to 1:13 000. Gelofusine is stable for 5 years at room temperature and does not contain a preservative. It does not interfere with blood grouping or cross-matching.

19. **With regard to antiarrhythmic agents:**
    A. oral amiodarone has an elimination half-life of approximately 1 month.
    B. lignocaine is effective after oral administration.
    C. sotalol prolongs the effective refractory period.
    D. the usual loading dose of quinidine is 1 mg/kg intravenously.
    E. phenytoin is a negative inotropic agent.

20. **Midazolam:**
    A. is water soluble at low pH due to opening of the benzodiazepine ring.
    B. causes anterograde amnesia.
    C. binds allosterically to γ-aminobutyric acid (GABA) receptors.
    D. has no active metabolites.
    E. has an elimination half-life of approximately 2 hours.

19. ACE

In the Vaughan Williams electrophysiological classification, class I agents block the fast sodium channel and are differentiated by prolongation (class Ia), shortening (class Ib) or no effect (class Ic) on the effective refractory period. Quinidine (class Ia) is invariably administered orally 300–600 mg q.d.s. because the intravenous route may cause severe hypotension. Lignocaine, tocainide and mexiletine are class Ib agents and are most effective in treating ventricular arrhythmias; lignocaine is ineffective orally because of low oral bioavailability due to high first pass metabolism. Class II agents are β-blockers and slow the rate of spontaneous diastolic depolarization. Class III agents prolong the effective refractory period and include amiodarone and sotalol. Class IV agents are the slow calcium channel blockers. Phenytoin (a class Ib agent), when given intravenously, can cause hypotension.

20. ABCE

The group characteristics of benzodiazepines are that they are water insoluble, have long half-lives of elimination, active metabolites and variable patient response. Their clinical actions include anterograde amnesia, sedation, anxiolysis, hypnosis and anticonvulsant activity. Midazolam has a novel open/closed ring structure conferring water solubility in the ampoule at pH 3.5 (open) and lipid solubility at pH 7.4 (closed); the lipid-soluble form has a pK_a of 6.2. Midazolam has a similar volume of distribution to diazepam (100 l) but a clearance 30 times higher, giving an elimination half-life of 2 hours. One metabolite, α-hydroxymidazolam, has sedative activity but is rapidly conjugated in the liver. The metabolite is likely to contribute to the clinical action only after long infusions of the parent compound. Benzodiazepines bind allosterically to the $GABA_A$ receptor and increase the activity of the endogenous ligand in opening the associated chloride channel. It appears that there are subtypes of GABA receptors, which may explain the differing clinical effects of the members of this group of drugs.

21. **Propofol:**
    A. is a weak organic acid with a pK_a of 11.
    B. contains Cremophor EL as the commercial solvent.
    C. is synergistic with alfentanil.
    D. is an effective analgesic.
    E. requires a blood concentration of approximately 12–14 µg/ml for induction of anaesthesia in unpremedicated patients.

21. **AC**

Propofol (2,6-diisopropylphenol) is a weak acid with a high pK_a, resulting in a large fraction of unionized, lipid-soluble drug at pH 7.4. Its water solubility is poor and it was initially presented in the solvent Cremophor EL. However this solvent causes a high incidence of anaphylactoid reactions. The drug is now presented commercially in a preparation containing glycerol, soybean oil, purified egg phosphatide, sodium hydroxide and water. It is believed that the solvent lipid load was the cause of death in several children following high infusion rates of propofol for several days in intensive care units. In unpremedicated patients, the effective blood concentration for induction of anaesthesia is approximately 3.5–3.9 µg/ml. The effective blood concentration to abolish response to surgery is influenced greatly by the blood concentration of co-administered opioid. Work with target-controlled infusions of alfentanil and propofol have demonstrated synergy, rather than a simple additive effect. The blood level of propofol (as sole agent) required to prevent movement to incision is 10–15 µg/ml.

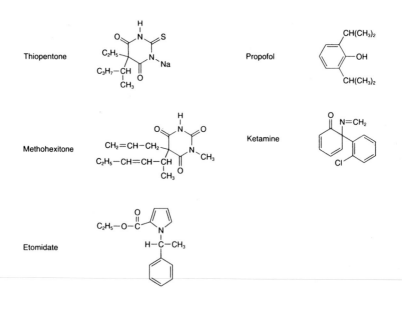

22. **With regard to opioids administered via the epidural space:**
    A. urinary retention is relatively common.
    B. low-dose naloxone alleviates pruritus without modifying analgesia.
    C. biphasic respiratory depression may occur.
    D. lipid solubility affects speed of onset.
    E. morphine is the agent of choice.

23. **Topical amethocaine gel:**
    A. is an ester.
    B. is available clinically in a 10% solution.
    C. is not licensed for use in neonates.
    D. is used topically for awake bronchoscopies.
    E. causes vasoconstriction which may make venous cannulation difficult.

24. **Phenol:**
    A. is used to inject haemorrhoids.
    B. causes skin necrosis.
    C. is an irritant to the eye.
    D. is injected as a 10% solution to destroy nerves.
    E. is useful in the treatment of psoriasis.

22. **ABCD**

The risk of respiratory depression appears to be dose related. Virtually all opioids have been reputed to cause delayed respiratory depression but morphine is associated with the highest incidence, approximately 1%. Other complications include pruritus (28–100%), nausea (30–100%) and urinary retention (15–90%). Again, morphine has the highest incidence of these side-effects and fentanyl the lowest; this is probably because the high lipid solubility of fentanyl binds the opioid at spinal cord level and little free drug is available in the cerebrospinal fluid (CSF) for rostral spread to the medulla.

23. **AC**

Topical amethocaine gel is available as a 4% solution to be applied to the limbs for local anaesthesia enabling venous cannulation to be painless, although it is not licensed for use in neonates. Application times of 30–45 min are recommended and surface anaesthesia may persist for 4 hours after a single application. Unlike EMLA cream, amethocaine causes local vasodilatation; slight oedema and itching may also be noticeable. Amethocaine is too toxic to be used in the airway, but is used as a topical solution in the eye. It is an ester local anaesthetic and is metabolized very rapidly by plasma cholinesterase. When applied to intact skin, the bioavailability is 15% with a mean absorption and elimination half-life of 1.2 hours. The main metabolite is butylaminobenzoic acid (BABA).

24. **ABCD**

Phenol is a weak acid with both bactericidal and neurolytic properties available in various preparations. For neurolytic therapy, 5–10% aqueous solutions are used and it may be mixed with glycerol to produce hyperbaric solutions for intrathecal use as well. The neurolytic effect is more pronounced on small $A\delta$ and C fibres which conduct pain, rather than the larger motor fibres. A 5% phenol solution in almond oil is used to inject haemorrhoids. Great care must be taken to avoid accidental splashes to the skin or eye.

25. **In standard clinical dosage, thiopentone:**
    A. has a pH of 10.5 in 2.5% solution.
    B. is 95% plasma protein bound.
    C. is metabolized at 10–15% per hour.
    D. has a pK_a of 9.1.
    E. contains 10 carbon atoms.

26. **The following are prodrugs:**
    A. enalapril.
    B. diamorphine.
    C. digitoxin.
    D. L-dopa.
    E. losartan.

27. **Drugs undergoing ester hydrolysis include:**
    A. pethidine.
    B. esmolol.
    C. procaine.
    D. aspirin.
    E. diamorphine.

25. AC

Barbituric acid is formed from urea and malonic acid and has no hypnotic activity. The first barbiturate was synthesized in 1903 and thiopentone was first administered in 1934. Thiopentone is 5-ethyl,5′-methylbutyl-thiobarbituric acid; it is 80–85% protein bound with a pK_a of 7.6, giving 61% unionized at pH 7.4. The dry powder in the ampoule is stored in an atmosphere of nitrogen and contains 6% sodium carbonate to give a pH of 10.5 in solution, increasing the solubility of the drug. Metabolism is by removal of the S atom to give pentobarbitone, oxidation to thiopentone carboxylic acid and cleavage of the ring. It contains 11 carbon atoms (see Paper 2 question 21).

26. ABD

Prodrugs are inactive or poorly active drugs that are metabolized to active substances. A number of ACE inhibitors (but not captopril) are prodrugs, e.g. enalapril-enalaprilat. Often prodrugs are used because of a desirable pharmacokinetic property; for example, diamorphine has a lipid solubility 200 times greater than that of morphine. However, the acetyl on the 3 position of the phenanthrene ring prevents binding of diamorphine to the μ receptor. Action of plasma cholinesterase produces the active metabolite 6-acetylmorphine. The prodrug dopa is administered orally together with a peripheral dopa decarboxylase inhibitor, ensuring high levels of the metabolite dopamine in the central nervous system (CNS). Digitoxin is the main glycoside from *Digitalis purpurea*, whereas digoxin comes from *Digitalis lanata*. Losartan is an angiotensin II receptor antagonist.

27. ABCDE

Esterases are found in plasma, red cells, liver, kidney, brain and intestinal mucosa. The generic term esterase includes choline and non-choline esterases. With some drugs, ester hydrolysis represents the sole metabolic pathway, e.g. suxamethonium, diamorphine and aspirin. In others it is an alternative pathway, e.g. atracurium.

28. **Pharmacokinetic drug interactions occur between the following:**
    A. non-depolarizing muscle relaxants and volatile anaesthetic agents.
    B. cimetidine and lignocaine.
    C. fentanyl and inhalational induction of anaesthesia.
    D. morphine and oral temazepam.
    E. atracurium and labetalol.

29. **Botulinum toxin:**
    A. is highly infectious.
    B. is derived from a plant mould.
    C. binds to the presynaptic membrane of the neuromuscular junction.
    D. has no beneficial clinical effects.
    E. causes direct muscle paralysis.

30. **Agents that remain largely in the intravascular space after intravenous administration include:**
    A. inulin.
    B. heparin.
    C. indocyanine green.
    D. hydroxyethyl starch (HES).
    E. warfarin.

28. BCD

Pharmacokinetic interactions are those in which one drug affects the free blood or tissue concentration of the other. They may be beneficial or detrimental. Interactions include delayed or accelerated absorption, alteration in protein binding, or altered distribution, metabolism or elimination. Fentanyl reduces alveolar minute ventilation and slows induction of anaesthesia with an inhalational agent. Morphine impairs gastric emptying and delays the onset of peak blood concentration of orally administered drugs. Cimetidine causes numerous interactions with drugs eliminated by hepatic metabolism through inhibition of hepatic microsomal function and reduction in hepatic blood flow. **A** is a pharmacodynamic interaction and **E** is not, as far as we know, a described drug interaction.

29. C

Botulinum toxin type A is a protein produced by *Clostridium botulinum* and is the most potent bacterial toxin known. It should be used within 1 hour of reconstitution and is not infectious. It binds to the presynaptic membrane of the neuromuscular junction and prevents acetylcholine release, causing neuromuscular blockade. In small doses it is a useful treatment of hemifacial spasm and blepharospasm. Muscles injected with the toxin become weak 2–20 days after injection and usually recover in 2–4 months, because of growth of new terminal axons.

30. BCDE

To remain within the circulating blood volume, molecules must be either very large (HES) or highly protein bound (warfarin, indocyanine green), or both (heparin). Glomerular filtration will, in general, filter molecules with molecular weight < 60 000. Thus gelofusine (30 000) does not remain in the intravascular space but starch solutions with a mean molecular weight > 200 000 will. Indocyanine green has been used as an indicator for cardiac output calculations.

31. **The following are true:**
    A. the *a* wave of the jugular venous pulse (JVP) coincides with the fourth heart sound (if present).
    B. the P–R interval of the ECG represents the duration of atrial systole.
    C. the T wave of the ECG ends at the time of aortic valve closure.
    D. the *c* wave of the JVP coincides with isovolumetric contraction of the right ventricle.
    E. the resting membrane potential of a single sinoatrial node cell is about 60 mV.

31. ABCD

The P wave of the ECG represents depolarization of the atria, and the QRS complex represents depolarization of the ventricles. Whilst repolarization of the atria is lost within the QRS complex and cannot be seen, repolarization of the ventricles is represented by the ST segment and T wave. Occasionally U waves are seen, which probably represent slow repolarization of the papillary muscles. A fourth heart sound is due to atrial contraction. The normal resting membrane potential is $-70\,mV$.

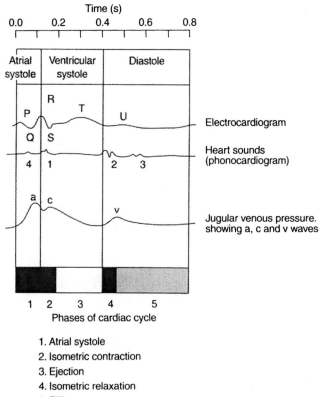

1. Atrial systole
2. Isometric contraction
3. Ejection
4. Isometric relaxation
5. Filling

32. **Diffusion across the alveolus into pulmonary vessels:**
    A. is quicker for oxygen than carbon dioxide.
    B. is quicker for carbon dioxide than nitrous oxide.
    C. is quicker for halothane than oxygen.
    D. is quicker for nitrous oxide than nitrogen.
    E. is quicker for carbon dioxide than carbon monoxide.

33. **Myocardial muscle differs from skeletal muscle in that myocardial muscle:**
    A. has a longer refractory period.
    B. can incur a greater oxygen debt.
    C. can metabolize lactic acid.
    D. contains no glycogen.
    E. contains no myosin.

34. **Systemic effects of hypercarbia include:**
    A. increase in the pain threshold.
    B. hypertension.
    C. sweating.
    D. vasoconstriction.
    E. bradycardia.

32. BCD

Diffusion is dependent upon the following factors: concentration difference (c); molecular weight (MW); cross-sectional area (XA); and thickness of the membrane (t). These factors are incorporated into an equation as follows:

$$\text{diffusion } \alpha \frac{c}{\sqrt{MW}} \times \frac{XA}{t}$$

Carbon dioxide and carbon monoxide diffuse rapidly, followed by nitrous oxide, nitrogen and inhalational agents and then oxygen.

33. AC

Cardiac muscle is similar to skeletal muscle in that they both contain myosin, troponin, actin and tropomyosin, but there is a longer refractory period after conduction through cardiac muscle, otherwise tetany (with disastrous consequences) could ensue. Normally cardiac muscle metabolism is aerobic with less than 1% being anaerobic, but in times of hypoxia up to 10% may become anaerobic. If metabolism is totally anaerobic then the energy liberated is not sufficient to sustain ventricular contraction. After a meal, cardiac muscle will metabolize pyruvate and lactate, and during periods of starvation it can metabolize fats.

34. BC

Hypercarbia results in a bounding pulse, sweating, vasodilatation, a shift in the oxygen–haemoglobin dissociation curve to the right and a reduction in the pain threshold. Modest levels of hypercarbia may be associated with positive inotropy, possibly through increased sympathetic nerve discharge and release of catecholamines, often resulting in arrhythmias. Hypercarbia causes respiratory stimulation and an increase in cerebral blood flow.

35. **Compared with extracellular fluid, intracellular fluid contains higher concentrations of:**
    A. bicarbonate.
    B. phosphate.
    C. calcium.
    D. magnesium.
    E. protein.

36. **The following are true regarding magnesium:**
    A. it is the most abundant intracellular cation.
    B. minimum adult daily needs are approximately 100 mmol.
    C. gastrointestinal absorption of magnesium is increased in the presence of parathyroid hormone.
    D. reduction in serum levels leads to tetany.
    E. magnesium causes vasodilatation.

37. **Regarding the work of breathing:**
    A. the majority is due to airways resistance.
    B. the elastic energy of the thoracic cage reduces some of the work of breathing.
    C. work of breathing is increased in congestive cardiac failure.
    D. work of breathing is reduced in emphysema.
    E. it is calculated by integrating pressure–volume curves.

35. BDE

	Intracellular fluid (mmol/l except*)	Extracellular fluid (mmol/l except *)
Sodium	10	140
Potassium	150	5
Calcium	1	2.5
Magnesium	13	1.5
Chloride	5	105
Protein	60	15
Bicarbonate	10	25
Phosphate	50	1
pH	7.0*	7.4*

36. CDE

Magnesium is the second most abundant intracellular cation following potassium. Hypomagnesaemia exists when the plasma level falls below 0.8 mmol/l and may result in confusion, tetany, ataxia and ultimately convulsions. Normal daily intake is approximately 12 mmol. Magnesium is utilized within enzyme systems, is required for normal neuromuscular function and causes direct vasodilatation. This latter effect is the rationale for the use of magnesium infusions to control hypertension in pre-eclampsia. The commonest causes of hypomagnesaemia are severe diarrhoea and pancreatitis.

37. BCE

The total work of breathing consists of elastic work (65%) and non-elastic work, i.e. airways resistance (30%) and viscous resistance (5%). The work required to inflate the whole system is less than that to inflate the lungs alone because of the elastic energy of the thoracic wall. Work of breathing is increased in acute asthma, congestive cardiac failure and chronic obstructive pulmonary disease.

38. **Regarding respiratory dead space:**
    A. anatomical dead space is calculated using the Bohr equation.
    B. physiological dead space is that volume of the respiratory tract not eliminating carbon dioxide.
    C. in healthy adults, physiological and anatomical dead space values are similar.
    D. anatomical dead space is reduced in the elderly.
    E. physiological dead space is measured using the nitrogen washout test.

39. **Functions of the kidney include secretion of:**
    A. ADH (vasopressin).
    B. renin.
    C. erythropoietin.
    D. active vitamin D.
    E. atrial natriuretic peptide (ANP).

38. BC

Anatomical dead space is the volume of the conducting airways, whereas physiological dead space is the volume of the respiratory tract not eliminating carbon dioxide and therefore consists of anatomical dead space *and* alveolar dead space. The most common way to estimate anatomical dead space is by use of Fowler's method (a single-breath nitrogen washout); the patient takes a single deep breath of 100% oxygen and exhales to residual volume with nitrogen being measured. Anatomical dead space is often increased in the elderly due to dilatation of the airways. Physiological dead space is calculated from the Bohr equation, which is the ratio of arterial carbon dioxide minus the mean mixed expired carbon dioxide divided by the arterial carbon dioxide. Physiological dead space is increased with the use of positive end-expiratory pressure (PEEP) and controlled ventilation.

39. BCD

Functions of the kidney include production and secretion of renin and erythropoietin. Deoxycholecalciferol is oxygenated to cholecalciferol (active vitamin D) in the kidney, whilst ADH and ANP both act in the kidney but are not secreted by it.

40. **The following cause a shift in the oxygen–haemoglobin dissociation curve to the right:**
    A. hypothermia.
    B. rise in 2,3-diphosphoglycerate (2,3-DPG).
    C. carboxyhaemoglobin.
    D. acidosis.
    E. fetal haemoglobin.

40. BD

The oxygen–haemoglobin dissociation curve relates percentage saturation of the oxygen-carrying power of haemoglobin to the partial pressure of arterial oxygen. It is sigmoid shaped because when one haem unit combines with oxygen it increases the affinity of the second haem unit for oxygen and so on, so that the affinity of haemoglobin for the fourth oxygen molecule is many times that for the first. The curve is shifted to the right, i.e. the partial pressure of arterial oxygen is higher for a given saturation, by the following:

> increase in 2,3-DPG, a substance with a half-life of 6 hours produced from the Embden–Meyerhof glycolysis pathway – this occurs in chronic anaemia and ascent to high altitude;
> acidosis; and
> rise in temperature.

The curve is shifted to the left by the opposite of the above, and by fetal haemoglobin and carboxyhaemoglobin.

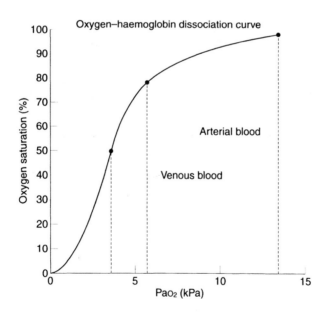

41. **Respiratory changes associated with liver failure include:**
    A. pleural effusions.
    B. arteriovenous shunts.
    C. impaired diaphragmatic movement.
    D. respiratory alkalosis.
    E. tension pneumothorax.

42. **Severe liver disease results in impaired production of:**
    A. albumin.
    B. α_1-acid glycoprotein.
    C. vitamin K.
    D. prothrombin.
    E. clotting factor VIII.

43. **A fixed, low cardiac output is associated with:**
    A. mitral stenosis.
    B. hypertrophic obstructive cardiomyopathy.
    C. aortic stenosis.
    D. ventricular septal defect (VSD).
    E. pericardial effusion.

41.   ABC

Changes in liver failure include the following.

Hypoxia due to arteriovenous shunts, sympathetic pleural effusions, raised diaphragm due to ascites, ventilation–perfusion mismatch due to overall increases in pulmonary blood flow.

Respiratory stimulation due to excessive ammonia production, which may result in hypocarbia.

A rise in serum 2,3-DPG causes a shift in the oxygen–haemoglobin dissociation curve to the right, resulting in reduced affinity of haemoglobin for oxygen and increased uptake of oxygen by the tissues; this mechanism counteracts some of the adverse effects mentioned above.

42.   AD

Severe liver disease results in the impaired production of albumin and all the clotting factors except factor VIII (produced by the reticuloendothelial system). There is increased production of α_1-acid glycoprotein, which may affect the plasma protein binding of drugs such as the amide-type local anaesthetics. Vitamin K is a fat-soluble vitamin and is not produced by the liver.

43.   ABCE

A fixed, low cardiac output describes the situation where the measured cardiac output is low and is not increased substantially by chronotropes or inotropes. The conditions that most commonly cause this are restrictive valvular disease, hypertrophic obstructive cardiomyopathy and pericardial effusion. A VSD may result in a hyperdynamic circulation.

44. **The tests required in the UK to establish brainstem death:**
  A. require an electroencephalograph (EEG) beforehand.
  B. may only be performed if the core temperature is 37°C.
  C. include absent ventilation in the presence of hypercarbia.
  D. require the absence of spinal reflexes.
  E. are often performed by a member of the transplant team.

44.   **C**

Brainstem death tests are usually performed on two separate occasions within a few hours of each other, although there are no specific time limits required (and the legal requirement stipulates only one test needs to be performed). They are performed by doctors with at least 5 years experience post qualification who must not be members of the transplant team. There must be a clinical diagnosis (or strong suspicion) for the cause of brainstem death. All patients, without exception, are unresponsive and ventilated. Drug causes, metabolic abnormalities, hypoxia and hypothermia (core temperature must be > 35°C) should all have been excluded before the tests are started. No EEG is required and spinal reflexes may still be present (which is why brain-dead patients are often paralysed during organ procurement). The tests performed are as follows.

Confirm absent cranial nerve reflexes: light, corneal, cough, gag and pain.

Confirm doll's eye movements and negative caloric tests (no eye movement when ice-cold water is poured into the ears).

Confirm no ventilatory response to hypercarbia. The patient is oxygenated for 10 min, often with some dead space volume added to the breathing circuit to allow the partial pressure of arterial carbon dioxide to rise. Arterial blood gases are taken to ensure that the patient has a normal arterial oxygen level and a suction catheter is inserted into the endotracheal tube and oxygen insufflated for 10 min whilst the patient is disconnected from the ventilator. At the end of this time another arterial sample is withdrawn to ensure that the arterial carbon dioxide level is at least 6.7 kPa. If there is no ventilatory response during this time and all the above tests have been performed, then the patient is diagnosed as suffering from irreversible brainstem death.

45. **A patient tells you that they bruise easily, but a full blood count, prothrombin time (PT), activated partial thromboplastin time (APTT) and bleeding time are all normal. The following may be the cause:**
   A. the patient is taking steroids.
   B. the patient is taking aspirin.
   C. the patient is elderly.
   D. the patient has Osler–Weber–Rendu syndrome.
   E. the patient has multiple myeloma.

46. **A third heart sound may be heard in the following conditions:**
   A. mitral stenosis.
   B. right ventricular failure.
   C. constrictive pericarditis.
   D. aortic stenosis.
   E. mitral regurgitation.

47. **In a normal unclothed adult, heat loss occurs through the following ways:**
   A. 40% through respiration.
   B. 30% through conduction.
   C. 30% through radiation.
   D. 30% through evaporation.
   E. 30% through convection.

45. **ACD**

There are four types of abnormal bleeding as shown in the table.

	Platelet count	Bleeding time	PT	APTT
Thrombocytopenia	Decreased	Increased	Normal	Normal
Abnormal platelet function	Normal	Increased	Normal	Normal
Coagulation disorders	Normal	Normal	Increased	Increased
Vascular bleeding disorders	Normal	Normal	Normal	Normal

A vascular bleeding disorder may be diagnosed if all four tests are normal and may be due to one of the following:

congenital: Osler–Weber–Rendu disease, characterized by multiple telangiectasia especially of the lips, nose and gastrointestinal tract

acquired ('the six Ss'): simple bleeding (i.e. unknown cause), senile bleeding (i.e. old age), scurvy (lack of vitamin C), steroid use, Henoch–Schönlein purpura, sepsis.

46. **BCE**

A third heart sound is due to rapid ventricular filling and may occur in the following situations:

it may be normal in people up to the age of 30
mitral or tricuspid regurgitation
left or right ventricular failure
cardiomyopathy
constrictive pericarditis
pulmonary embolus.

47. **CDE**

Temperature homeostasis is important in the body for the normal function of enzyme reactions, neural function, blood flow and muscle contractility. Heat in the body is produced from digestion of food, metabolism and exercise. The body loses heat in the following ways:

skin: radiation 30%, evaporation 30%, convection 30%
respiration 10%
urine and faeces (minimal amounts).

48. **Compared with adults, neonates:**
    A. breathe through their mouths.
    B. have a reduced basal metabolic rate per square metre of body surface area.
    C. are resistant to the effects of opioids.
    D. have a less compliant chest wall.
    E. demonstrate right-axis deviation on the ECG.

49. **Within the adrenal gland:**
    A. catecholamines are secreted by the adrenal medulla.
    B. dopamine is a precursor of noradrenaline.
    C. the cortex is derived embryologically from the neural crest.
    D. bilateral adrenalectomy results in death due to loss of medullary function.
    E. phaeochromocytomas are derived from the adrenal cortex.

48. **E**

Compared with adults, neonates (infants up to the age of 1 month) exhibit the physiological differences listed in the table.

Cardiovascular
Increased blood volume (80 ml/kg)
Relatively increased cardiac output (primarily due to increased heart rate)
Right-axis deviation on the ECG
Haemoglobin 18 g/dl at birth (reducing to a low of 11 g/dl at 6 weeks of age as fetal haemoglobin is exchanged for adult haemoglobin)
Lower systemic blood pressure

Respiratory
Relatively large head and tongue, greater jaw angle, high anterior larynx, U-shaped epiglottis and the narrowest part of airway is subglottic
Nasal breathers
High respiratory rate
Impaired response to hypoxia and hypercarbia
Increased resistance to breathing
Compliant chest wall

Neurological
Incomplete myelination until 1 year old
Spinal cord ends lower (L3,4)
Sensitive to CNS depressants

Others
Immature kidneys
Increased surface area to weight ratio (70% of heat loss is due to radiation) and tendency to develop hypothermia
Brown fat metabolism
Tendency to hypoglycaemia and hypocalcaemia

49. **AB**

The adrenal medulla is derived from the neural crest and secretes catecholamines (dopamine, adrenaline and noradrenaline), whilst the cortex secretes cortisol (glucocorticoid), aldosterone (mineralocorticoid) and small amounts of testosterone and oestradiol; 90% of phaeochromocytomas are derived from the adrenal medulla whilst the remaining 10% are located outside the adrenal gland. Following bilateral adrenalectomy, replacement of glucocorticoid and mineralocorticoid are achieved by hydrocortisone 10–30 mg and fludrocortisone 0.1–0.2 mg daily.

50. **The following are essential trace elements:**
    A. copper.
    B. magnesium.
    C. arsenic.
    D. phosphate.
    E. zinc.

51. **Alcoholic patients are more likely than normal patients to suffer from:**
    A. hypothermia during anaesthesia.
    B. increased blood loss during anaesthesia.
    C. hyperglycaemia.
    D. impaired stress response.
    E. postoperative infections.

52. **The stretch reflex in the gastrocnemius muscle:**
    A. is an example of negative feedback.
    B. is related to the degree of stretch.
    C. has a rapid monosynaptic component.
    D. shows reciprocal inhibition of antagonist muscle groups.
    E. is inhibited at high levels of tension in the muscle.

50. ACE
Trace elements that are essential for life are listed in the table.

Zinc	Iron
Iodine	Molybdenum
Nickel	Silicon
Copper	Vanadium
Manganese	Selenium
Arsenic	Chromium
Fluorine	Cobalt

Trace elements are found in tissues in minute amounts and deficiency is rare unless associated with other dietary problems. Toxicity due to the presence of excessive trace elements may occur, e.g. copper in Wilson's disease and iron in haemochromatosis.

51. ABDE
Alcoholics have acute and chronic physical and mental problems of importance to anaesthetists.

Acute problems	Chronic problems
Impaired airway reflexes	Cardiac arrhythmias and cardiomyopathy
Impaired ability to vasoconstrict in response to blood loss	Liver disease
Difficult to assess clinically	Autonomic neuropathy
Risk of vomiting increased	Impaired clotting
Hypoglycaemia and hypothermia	Peripheral neuropathy

52. ABCDE
When an innervated skeletal muscle is stretched it contracts and the stretch reflex in the gastrocnemius muscle (the ankle reflex) is an example of a monosynaptic reflex (similar to the knee, triceps and masseter reflexes). Up to a certain point, the harder a muscle is stretched the stronger is the contraction, until the stretch is so great that the contraction suddenly ceases and the muscle relaxes; this is termed the inverse stretch reflex or autogenic inhibition. There is also negative feedback and reciprocal inhibition of antagonist muscle groups whereby the sensory nerves within the stretched muscle spindles cause postsynaptic inhibition of motor nerves to the antagonist muscles.

53. **The following infections may be transmitted through blood transfusions:**
    A. tuberculosis.
    B. syphilis.
    C. brucellosis.
    D. diphtheria.
    E. malaria.

54. **The following are true of pulmonary dynamics:**
    A. total compliance is maximal at functional residual capacity (FRC).
    B. prolonged anaesthesia results in a reduction in lung compliance.
    C. dynamic compliance is usually measured at the end of inspiration during intermittent positive pressure ventilation.
    D. an area of unventilated lung receives a greater blood flow than normally ventilated lung.
    E. normal total compliance is $100\,\text{ml/cmH}_2\text{O}$ [1 litre/kPa].

53. BCE

Blood may transmit the following infections:

bacterial: brucellosis, syphilis

viral: hepatitis A–F, human T-cell leukaemia (HTLV) 1 and 2, HIV, cytomegalovirus (CMV), glandular fever and parvovirus

parasitic: toxoplasmosis, trypanosomiasis, malaria, *Babesia microti*

Blood donors in the UK are aged 18–65, are voluntary and unpaid and may give blood two to three times a year. They should weigh at least 50 kg and be in good general health, not anaemic, pregnant or have a malignancy (except fully treated locally invasive tumours, e.g. rodent ulcers). They should not have travelled to a malaria-infested geographical area within the previous 3 months. Blood taken from donors is tested for haemoglobin level (using copper sulphate), sterility, blood grouping, red blood cell antibodies and HLA typed. Blood is tested for the presence of antibodies to HIV, TPHA (syphilis) and selected blood for antibodies to CMV and is also antigen tested for hepatitis B and C.

Barbara, J.A.J. & Contreras, M. (1990) Infectious complications of blood transfusion: bacteria and parasites. *BMJ* **300**, 386–389.
Barbara, J.A.J. & Contreras, M. (1990) Infectious complications of blood transfusion: viruses. *BMJ* **300**: 450–453.

54. BE

Compliance varies with lung volume and is greatest at a lung volume 1 litre greater than the FRC, and lowest at total lung capacity. Static compliance is measured when no air is flowing; dynamic compliance, measured when air is flowing, includes airway resistance to flow. Normal static values for lung and chest wall combined are $100 \, ml/cmH_2O$ (1 litre/kPa). Hypoxic pulmonary vasoconstriction reduces blood flow to areas of lung with poor ventilation.

55. **The difference between alveolar and arterial partial pressure of oxygen in normal subjects breathing room air is:**
    A. usually 2.5–3.5 kPa.
    B. contributed to by shunting of blood from bronchial to pulmonary veins.
    C. contributed to by the draining of thebesian veins into the right ventricle.
    D. likely to be increased by collapse of the right upper lobe.
    E. likely to be reduced by a fall in cardiac output.

56. **Stomach emptying is stimulated by:**
    A. atropine.
    B. dopamine.
    C. salbutamol.
    D. small bowel distension.
    E. propranolol.

57. **The following are true regarding the Valsalva manoeuvre:**
    A. it is a forced expiration against a closed glottis.
    B. it is associated with the development of $400\,cmH_2O$ pressure.
    C. it initially causes an increase in venous return.
    D. a square wave response is seen in autonomic neuropathy.
    E. a blocked response is seen in patients taking β-adrenergic antagonists.

55. BD

Oxygen diffuses freely across the alveolar membrane, and alveolar and end-pulmonary capillary oxygen tensions are equal. The difference between alveolar and arterial oxygen levels in normal people is caused by venous admixture, due to a small amount of deoxygenated blood mixing with oxygenated blood in the arterial system as follows: draining of thebesian veins from the heart into the left ventricle and shunting of blood from bronchial to pulmonary veins. This venous admixture is often termed 'physiological shunt' and has a value of 2%, i.e. the difference between alveolar and arterial oxygen tensions can be explained *as though* 2% of the cardiac output is not being oxygenated.

56. E

When food enters the stomach, the stomach relaxes and peristaltic waves mix the food and squirt it into the duodenum at a controlled rate. Stomach emptying is increased by the following:

cholinergic effects (vagotomy will reduce the rate of emptying)
reduced sympathetic effects
antidopaminergic effects
food in the stomach (carbohydrates leave the stomach more quickly than proteins, which leave more quickly than fatty foods).

57. AE

The Valsalva manoeuvre is a forced expiration against a closed glottis and approximately $40\,cmH_2O$ pressure is developed. Because of the development of raised intrathoracic pressure the systemic blood pressure initially increases (transiently) due to transmission of the increased intrathoracic pressure to the aorta. The pressure then drops due to reduction in the venous return and consequent fall in cardiac output. Due to inhibition of the baroreceptors a reflex tachycardia and increase in peripheral vascular resistance results until the blood pressure returns to normal. When the Valsalva is stopped, there is a sudden increase in the venous return and the blood pressure rises. This is sensed by the baroreceptors, and a reflex bradycardia and reduction in peripheral vascular resistance occurs to bring the blood pressure back to normal. A square wave response in seen in heart failure and indicates inability to respond to heart rate changes, whilst a blocked response (absent heart rate changes) is seen in adrenergic blockade or autonomic neuropathy.

58. **Insulin:**
    A. is secreted by the B cells of the pancreas.
    B. inhibits liver glycogenolysis.
    C. inhibits lipolysis.
    D. is essential for glucose uptake within the CNS.
    E. has a half-life of approximately 5 min.

58. **ABCE**

Insulin is a peptide consisting of 51 amino acids arranged in two chains (A and B) linked by disulphide bridges and is derived from the cleavage of preproinsulin to proinsulin and then to insulin. Insulin has a half-life of 5 minutes, is secreted in amounts of up to 300 nmol daily by the B cells of the pancreas and may be measured in the blood (normal levels are up to 500 pmol/l) by radioimmunoassay. It is metabolized in the liver and kidney. Actions of insulin include:

  facilitating glucose uptake into most cells except red blood cells, brain (apart from the hypothalamus), gastrointestinal tract mucosa and renal tubules
  increasing protein and lipid synthesis
  glycogenesis in the liver and muscle.

59. **Regarding arginine vasopressin (ADH):**
    A. it is a peptide hormone.
    B. secretion is increased by exercise.
    C. secretion is increased by alcohol intake.
    D. the antidiuretic effect is due to an increase in permeability to water in the distal convoluted tubule and collecting duct.
    E. it causes hypertension when given in standard clinical dosage.

59. ABD

Arginine vasopressin (ADH) is a nonapeptide secreted by the posterior pituitary together with oxytocin (another nonapeptide). They are both neural hormones, i.e. hormones secreted into the circulation by nerve cells. ADH has a half-life of 18 min and there are three different receptor subtypes.

V_{1A} receptors are located on blood vessels and stimulation results in vasoconstriction. However, in normal clinical dosage there is not usually an increase in blood pressure because ADH also acts on the area postrema in the brain, resulting in a reduction in cardiac output that negates the vasoconstrictive effects.

V_{1B} receptors are located in the anterior pituitary and stimulation results in adrenocorticotrophic hormone (ACTH) secretion.

V_2 receptors are located in the kidney and stimulation results in antidiuresis; water enters the hypertonic interstitium of the renal pyramids, so that the urine becomes concentrated and reduced in volume.

The factors listed in the table cause an increase or decrease in ADH secretion.

Increase	Decrease
Reduced extracellular fluid	Increased extracellular fluid
Increased osmotic pressure	Reduced osmotic pressure
Stress and exercise	Alcohol
Morphine and nicotine	α-Adrenergic agonists
Prostaglandin E_2	
Angiotensin II	
Barbiturates and carbamazepine	
β-Adrenergic agonists	

60. **Normal requirements for total parenteral nutrition in an average sized adult include:**
    A. 10 g of protein per day.
    B. 2000–2500 kcal per day.
    C. 1 g of carbohydrate provides 9 kcal.
    D. a mixture of non-essential and essential free fatty acids.
    E. 100 g of fat per day.

61. **The following statements concern heat:**
    A. the specific heat capacity of a substance is the energy required to raise the temperature of 1 g of a substance by 1 K.
    B. the specific heat capacity of gases is greater than the specific heat capacity of liquids.
    C. the latent heat of vaporization is the amount of heat required to convert a unit mass of liquid into vapour without a change in temperature.
    D. the boiling point of any liquid is the temperature at which its saturated vapour pressure is equal to ambient pressure.
    E. highly volatile agents have a lower saturated vapour pressure than less volatile liquids.

60. BDE

The normal adult dietary intake consists of approximately 2500 kcal of which 300 g is from carbohydrate, 75 g is from protein and 100 g is from fat (where 1 g nitrogen (6.25 g protein) provides 25 kcal, 1 g carbohydrate provides 4 kcal and 1 g fat provides 9 kcal). The fat within the diet should consist of at least 50% as essential fatty acids and the protein should consist of at least 40% as essential amino acids. Malnutrition is defined by the ratio of actual body weight divided by ideal body weight or normal (premorbid) body weight; a ratio of less than 9/10 is defined as malnutrition. If this ratio is less than 8/10 then there is a definite increase in mortality and morbidity (impaired wound healing and infections). Diagnosis of malnutrition may be made from an accurate history and examination, including anthropometric measurements such as Harpenden skin fold measurement (posterior triceps of non-dominant arm is normally less than 13 mm in females and 10 mm in males). Blood tests which may indicate malnutrition include:

serum albumin ($< 30\,g/l$)
serum transferrin ($< 2\,g/l$)
serum prealbumin ($< 0.2\,g/l$)
serum retinol-binding protein ($< 0.1\,g/l$).

61. CD

The specific heat capacity of a substance is the energy required to raise the temperature of 1 kg of the substance by 1 K. The specific heat capacity of liquids is up to 1000 times greater than that of gases. Highly volatile agents have a lower boiling point and higher saturated vapour pressure (the vapour above the liquid is present in a higher concentration) than less volatile agents. The saturated vapour pressure is the maximum pressure that can be exerted by the vapour at a specific temperature and the rise of saturated vapour pressure with temperature is non-linear. When saturated vapour pressure equals atmospheric pressure the liquid "boils".

62. **The rate of infusion of a fluid through a giving set and intravenous cannula is directly proportional to:**
    A. viscosity of the fluid.
    B. venous back pressure.
    C. internal diameter of cannula.
    D. length of cannula.
    E. height of chamber in the giving set.

63. **The following relate to the venturi effect:**
    A. it relies on the Bernoulli principle.
    B. it utilizes the principle that a pressure gradient develops when a fluid or gas passes through a constriction.
    C. it states that there is an increase in pressure as a fluid passes through a constriction.
    D. the velocity of the fluid remains constant throughout.
    E. it is similar in principle to the Coanda effect.

62. CE

'Directly proportional' indicates that the flow of fluid increases with an increase in magnitude of the specified factor. The rate of infusion depends upon:

the height of the fluid chamber (directly)
back pressure from the veins (inversely)
length of the cannula (inversely)
internal diameter of the cannula (directly)
physical properties of the fluid being infused (inversely for viscosity).

63. AB

The Bernoulli principle describes gas flow through a tube incorporating a narrowed section. The gas flow will accelerate as it encounters the narrowing. Because the total energy must remain constant, as the gas accelerates the pressure falls. Equally, as the gas leaves the constriction back into the wider lumen the velocity falls and the pressure rises. The drop in pressure at the constriction can be utilized to entrain another gas; this entrainment will be at a constant rate as long as the velocity of the gas and the dimensions of the constriction remain constant; this is known as the venturi effect. The Coanda effect occurs when a jet of fluid or gas travels down a tube that bifurcates. If the tube divides equally into two branches the jet will pass down one or other side rather than split equally.

64. Nitrous oxide:

A. supports combustion.
B. was discovered by Joseph Priestley.
C. in hospitals is usually supplied from a large vacuum insulated container (VIC).
D. cylinders have a filling ratio of 0.7 in the UK.
E. is supplied at a pipeline pressure of 44 bar.

65. Thermistors:

A. produce a linear change in electrical resistance with change in temperature.
B. rely on a potential difference developing at the junction of two dissimilar metals.
C. are extremely fragile.
D. are a type of transducer.
E. demonstrate the Seebeck effect.

64. ABD

Nitrous oxide was discovered in 1772 by Joseph Priestley and first used as an anaesthetic by Wells in 1844 for a tooth extraction. It is a colourless sweet smelling gas obtained by heating ammonium nitrate to 240°C and removing impurities such as ammonia and nitric oxide. The boiling point is -88°C and the critical temperature is 36.5°C. It has a low blood:gas solubility coefficient of 0.47 and an oil:gas solubility coefficient of 1.4. It is non-flammable but does support combustion. In the UK it is supplied in blue cylinders containing liquid nitrous oxide at a pressure of 44 bar at 20°C. Pipeline supplies are from banks of cylinders with a pipeline pressure of 4 bar. Nitrous oxide is a strong analgesic but has weak anaesthetic properties with an MAC of 105%. Effects on the body include slight respiratory depression, little effect on the myocardium in healthy patients but in combination with volatile agents and in patients with reduced cardiovascular reserve it may depress myocardial function. It causes an increase in cerebral blood flow and raises intracranial pressure. Because it is some 30 times more soluble than nitrogen it causes expansion of gas-filled cavities. At the end of anaesthesia diffusion hypoxia may result unless a high inspired oxygen concentration is given. Prolonged exposure to nitrous oxide has been shown to inhibit methionine synthetase, which may lead to megaloblastic anaemia.

65. D

Thermistors are transducers (devices that convert one form of energy to another) used commonly to measure body temperature and which work on the principle that resistance in a metal oxide semiconductor falls with an increase in temperature. The relationship is an exponential one and so calibration may be difficult. Thermocouples (rather than thermistors) demonstrate the Seebeck effect: a voltage is produced at the junction of two different metal conductors and this voltage is proportional to temperature.

66. **Surface tension in a liquid is:**
   A. measured in kilopascals.
   B. due to mutual attraction between molecules.
   C. altered by changes in temperature.
   D. responsible for the formation of bubbles and droplets.
   E. directly proportional to its radius if a bubble is formed.

67. **Compared with nitrogen, helium has:**
   A. a lower density .
   B. a lower viscosity.
   C. a greater thermal conduction.
   D. a greater narcotic effect at high pressures.
   E. greater tissue solubility.

66. BCD

Surface tension (measured in newtons/metre or dynes/cm) results from tangential forces across the surface of a liquid. It is due to the mutual attraction between molecules in a liquid, which at the surface are only attracted inwards and so will contract to form the smallest surface area; this results in the formation of bubbles and droplets. The pressure (P) within a bubble is inversely proportional to its radius (r) and is given by the formula:

$$P = \frac{2T}{r}$$

where T is the surface tension.

67. AC

Helium is an inert gas supplied in brown cylinders at a pressure of 137 bar or mixed with 21% oxygen in black cylinders with white and brown quartered shoulders at 137 bar. Helium has a lower density than nitrogen but a higher viscosity, which means that it can be useful in upper airway obstruction where flow is turbulent and is influenced by the density of gases but of no use in lower airway obstruction where the flow is laminar and influenced by gas viscosity. When used in diving, the greater tissue solubility of nitrogen results in problems of bubbles of nitrogen forming in the blood if ascent is too rapid (decompression sickness or the 'bends'). Nitrogen also has a narcotic effect which is not seen with helium.

68. **With regard to ventilators:**
    A. constant pressure generators compensate well in patients with bronchospasm.
    B. constant flow generators compensate well for leaks in the breathing system.
    C. constant flow generators are suitable for patients with changing lung compliance.
    D. constant pressure generators deliver gases at a constant flow rate.
    E. the Blease Brompton Manley is of the bag squeezer type.

69. **The Magill breathing system:**
    A. is an example of a semi-open breathing system.
    B. has a rebreathing bag adjacent to the common gas outlet.
    C. is an example of a Mapleson A system.
    D. requires fresh gas flows equivalent to at least the patient's minute volume to prevent rebreathing during spontaneous respiration.
    E. has an expiratory valve at the patient end of the circuit.

68. C

Ventilators may be classified in a variety of ways as shown in the table.

Functional	Descriptive
Pressure or volume control	Mechanical thumbs
Inspiratory/expiratory cycling	Minute volume dividers
Pressure or flow generator	Bag squeezers
	Intermittent blowers

A constant flow generator presents a constant flow to the airway, whereas a constant pressure generator presents a constant pressure. In the latter device, lung compliance and airway resistance affect the actual flow of gas into the lungs. Constant flow generators compensate well for changes in compliance but poorly for leaks. The converse is true for constant pressure generators. The Blease Brompton Manley is a minute volume divider; the fresh gas flow enters and 'powers' the ventilator, which divides the minute volume into clinician-adjusted tidal volumes.

69. CE

The Magill breathing system is an example of a semi-closed Mapleson A breathing system. It has a reservoir bag (not rebreathing bag) and adjustable pressure limiting (APL) valve at the patient end of the system. It is very efficient for spontaneous ventilation because dead space gas is reused with the next breath, whilst alveolar gas is vented through the valve. Theoretically the fresh gas flow must be equal to the patient's alveolar ventilation to prevent rebreathing. However, the system is inefficient for positive pressure ventilation because squeezing the bag results in loss of fresh gas through the valve and fresh gas flows equal to two to three times the patient's minute ventilation are required to prevent rebreathing.

70. **Oxygen failure devices fitted to anaesthetic machines:**
    A. should sound for at least 4 s.
    B. may be electronically driven in new anaesthetic machines.
    C. must be linked to an antihypoxic gas cut-off device.
    D. should sound when the oxygen supply pressure falls to approximately 200 kPa.
    E. may be turned off when the machine is not in use.

71. **With regard to flowmeters:**
    A. rotameters work on the variable orifice principle.
    B. readings should be taken from the top of a ball bobbin flowmeter.
    C. oxygen flowmeters must be situated downstream of all other gas flowmeters.
    D. the use of certain types of ventilator may affect the calibration of the flowmeters.
    E. changes in temperature may produce significant inaccuracies.

70. CD

The features of an oxygen failure device are:

an audible alarm of at least 7 s duration triggered when the oxygen supply pressure falls to less than 200 kPa; the alarm sound should record 60 dB at 1 metre from the front of the anaesthetic machine;

the alarm must be powered by oxygen and it should not be possible to switch it off;

the delivery of other anaesthetic gases should be cut off (the machine usually opens to air);

the gas cut-off should not activate before the oxygen alarm has sounded;

the gas cut-off device and alarm cannot be reset until the oxygen pressure is greater than 200 kPa.

71. AD

The purpose of a flowmeter is to accurately control and quantitate the flow of gas through an anaesthetic machine. The flowmeter consists of a vertically tapered tube, a float and a control valve to adjust the gas flow. When gas enters the tube the float rises, allowing gas to flow in the space between the float and the wall of the tube. At low flow the gas flows through a narrow annulus and the resulting laminar flow is dependent upon the viscosity of the gas. At higher flow rates the gas flows through a much larger orifice and turbulent flow occurs, which is dependent upon the density of the gas. Each flowmeter must therefore be calibrated for a particular gas. Flow rates should be read from the top of a float or the middle of a ball bobbin. Causes of inaccuracy include:

the rotameter is not mounted completely vertical so that contact occurs between the float and the wall;

static electricity – to prevent this, the outside of the tube is sprayed with an antistatic agent and the inside of the tube is coated with a thin layer of conductor (usually gold);

dirt within the tube;

cracked flowmeter tube.

The oxygen flowmeter is traditionally situated to the left hand (upstream) side of the block of flowmeters but the oxygen is actually delivered downstream of the other gases.

72. **Scavenging systems for waste anaesthetic gases:**
    A. are generally designed to be high flow, low pressure systems.
    B. are usually passive.
    C. are fitted with 22-mm connectors.
    D. are colour coded yellow and green.
    E. usually feed directly into the hospital piped vacuum system.

73. **With regard to electrical supplies:**
    A. when wiring a plug the blue cable connects to neutral.
    B. ventricular fibrillation can result from a current as small as 75 mA passing through the body.
    C. the 'let go' threshold is about 15 mA.
    D. microshock of 15 μA applied directly to the heart can result in ventricular fibrillation.
    E. mains alternating supply in the UK is set at 500 Hz.

74. **With regard to pressure relief valves:**
    A. they are commonly used in anaesthetic breathing systems.
    B. the Heidbrink valve is an example.
    C. at equilibrium, the force exerted by the spring equals the force exerted by the gas within the breathing system.
    D. anaesthetic machines have a pressure relief valve of 350 kPa situated on the back bar.
    E. scavenging systems contain pressure relief valves.

72. A

Scavenging systems are designed to transport waste gases from the breathing system and discharge them at a safe location and should be available in any location where anaesthetic gases are being used. Systems may be active, whereby gas transport occurs due to negative pressure generated in the system, or passive, whereby transport occurs as a result of patient expiration. Active systems are able to cope with a much wider range of expiratory flow rates. Scavenging systems have specific 30-mm connectors to prevent incorrect connection within the breathing system, which has 15- or 22-mm connectors.

73. ABC

When wiring a plug the blue connects to neutral, the brown to live and yellow/green to earth. Mains electricity in the UK is 50 Hz, which happens to be particularly effective at producing ventricular fibrillation. When applied externally the threshold of feeling is a current of approximately 0.5 mA. Muscular contraction and inability to 'let go' of the source occurs at currents of 15 mA, whilst ventricular fibrillation occurs at currents of 75–100 mA. When applied directly to the heart much smaller currents of 100–150 µA can induce ventricular fibrillation, so-called 'microshock'. It is important that equipment connected to intracardiac catheters has an earth-free patient circuit to avoid these microcurrents; in practice this is achieved by using isolating transformers creating a fully floating circuit, which is designated as Class 3 equipment (Class 1 consists of equipment where the casing is earthed and Class 2 where all conducting wires within the equipment are double earthed).

74. ABCE

The Heidbrink valve is an example of an adjustable pressure relief valve commonly used in adult anaesthetic breathing systems. The anaesthetist is able to control the pressure within the breathing system by turning the valve, which controls the force in the spring below it. The spring force is balanced by the gas pressure and the area of the disc valve. The valve is set at a maximum pressure of 60 cmH$_2$O. The back bar of the anaesthetic machine is fitted with a pressure relief valve operating at 35 kPa, which protects the flowmeters from damage should the fresh gas outlet be occluded. Anaesthetic scavenging systems have pressure relief valves operating at relatively low pressures of 0.2–0.3 kPa.

75. **A fuel cell for measuring inspired oxygen concentrations:**
    A. is similar to a battery cell.
    B. has a potential difference between anode and cathode proportional to the oxygen concentration.
    C. usually has a gold anode.
    D. usually contains a potassium hydroxide electrolyte solution.
    E. works on the principle that oxygen is paramagnetic.

76. **The triservice apparatus contains:**
    A. one vaporizer.
    B. a self-inflating bag.
    C. a non-rebreathing valve.
    D. an oxygen cylinder.
    E. a face mask.

77. **The Lack circuit:**
    A. has fresh gas flowing through the inner tube.
    B. has an inner tube diameter of 15 mm.
    C. has an external diameter of 30 mm.
    D. has a reservoir bag mounted at the machine end.
    E. is efficient for spontaneous breathing.

75. ABD

A fuel cell for measuring oxygen concentrations is similar to a battery cell. Within the fuel cell the potential difference between the anode and cathode is proportional to the oxygen concentration. The fuel cell commonly has a lead anode and gold mesh cathode suspended in a potassium hydroxide solution. At the anode, electrons are released by the combination of hydroxyl ions with lead:

$$Pb + 2(OH^-) \rightarrow PbO + 2e^- + H_2O$$

The electrons combine with oxygen at the cathode:

$$O_2 + 4e^- + 2H_2O \rightarrow 4(OH^-)$$

The reaction is temperature sensitive, which is allowed for by use of a thermistor.

76. BCE

The triservice apparatus was designed for use in the field of combat, where there is no cylinder source of oxygen. It consists of a facemask with a non-rebreathing valve, tubing, a self-inflating bag, more tubing, two vaporizers (Oxford Miniature Vaporizers) and a further length of tubing which acts as an oxygen reservoir or can be connected to an oxygen source. In spontaneous respiration mode, the patient inspires air through the vaporizers and exhaled gases leave via the non-rebreathing valve, whilst in controlled ventilation mode the self-inflating bag is used.

77. CDE

The Lack system is a coaxial version of the Mapleson A and is therefore efficient for spontaneous respiration. It has an outer tube that is 30 mm in diameter and carries fresh gas to the patient, and an inner tube 14 mm in diameter which takes expired gases to the adjustable pressure limiting (APL) valve. Both the reservoir bag and the APL valve are situated at the machine end, making the circuit less cumbersome than the Magill circuit.

78. **Single-lumen Hickman catheters:**
    A. are usually made of silicone.
    B. are used for continuous venovenous haemofiltration.
    C. are usually inserted into the right internal jugular vein.
    D. may be a route for ventricular fibrillation due to 'micro-shock'.
    E. must be replaced every 4 weeks.

79. **The Humphrey ADE circuit:**
    A. has a valve that opens at a pressure of greater than 60 cmH$_2$O.
    B. requires a fresh gas flow in adults of at least 100 ml/kg per min in spontaneous respiration mode.
    C. is unsuitable for use in children.
    D. in spontaneous mode acts as a Bain breathing circuit.
    E. requires a fresh gas flow in adults of at least 100 ml/kg per min during positive-pressure ventilation.

80. **The Portex minitracheostomy:**
    A. has an internal diameter of 5 mm.
    B. uses the Seldinger technique for insertion.
    C. is inserted through the cricothyroid membrane.
    D. is 10 cm in length.
    E. may cause perforation of the oesophagus.

78. AD

Hickman central venous catheters are made of silicone or polyurethane and inserted into the subclavian vein (more comfortable for the patient than the internal jugular vein) by a Seldinger technique and then tunnelled under the skin to emerge near the axilla. They are usually inserted for long-term (several months) chemotherapy, parenteral nutrition or frequent venous blood sampling. All central venous catheters may cause microshock due to tiny electrical currents being directly transmitted to the myocardium. Venovenous haemofiltration requires a double-lumen wide-bore catheter.

79. A

The Humphrey ADE system is a versatile breathing circuit efficient for both spontaneous and controlled ventilation in both adults and children. The circuit can be changed by the movement of a lever from a Mapleson A during spontaneous respiration to an E during controlled ventilation so that the fresh gas flows required are as follows.

	Adult	Child
Spontaneous respiration	50–60 ml/kg per min	3 1/min
Controlled ventilation	70 ml/kg per min	3 1/min

80. CDE

The Portex minitracheostomy consists of a plastic tube (internal diameter 4 mm, length 10 cm) inserted into the trachea via the cricothyroid membrane. The tube is inserted using a scalpel blade and introducer (rather than a Seldinger technique) and the proximal end has a flange to secure the tube at the surface of the skin. It is useful for clearing airway secretions and may be used as a holding method to oxygenate the patient in failed intubation or ventilation situations. Significant complications of insertion include perforation of the oesophagus, haemorrhage and pneumothorax.

81. **Venturi-type face masks:**
    A. are examples of fixed-performance devices.
    B. require an oxygen flow rate of 15 l/min to produce a fraction of inspired oxygen (Fio_2) of 0.6.
    C. utilize the concept of rebreathing expired oxygen.
    D. include the MC mask.
    E. are contraindicated for use in patients dependent on hypoxic drive.

82. **The Penlon Nuffield 200 ventilator:**
    A. is a minute volume divider.
    B. is time cycled.
    C. is driven by oxygen from the common gas outlet.
    D. delivers a minimum tidal volume of 50 ml.
    E. cannot be used with a circle system.

81. **AB**

Venturi masks are fixed-performance or high air flow oxygen enrichment (HAFOE) devices which utilize the Bernoulli principle to entrain air mixed with an oxygen supply and deliver a fixed concentration to the patient. Six masks are available, all capable of delivering fixed concentrations of oxygen, as follows:

24% requires 2 l/min oxygen supply
28% requires 4 l/min oxygen supply
31% requires 6 l/min oxygen supply
35% requires 8 l/min oxygen supply
40% requires 10 l/min oxygen supply
60% requires 15 l/min oxygen supply

82. **BD**

The Nuffield Penlon 200 is a time-cycled flow generator. It is driven by oxygen from the compressed oxygen outlet and has inspired and expired time control dials and an inspiratory flow rate control knob. It can be used with several types of breathing systems including Bain, Humphrey ADE and the circle. In the adult mode the minimum tidal volume delivered is 50 ml, but if a Newton (paediatric) valve is added the ventilator changes to a time-cycled pressure generator capable of delivering tidal volumes of between 10 and 300 ml (depending on compliance) and is used for patients weighing less than 20 kg.

83. **The natural frequency of an arterial monitoring system is related to:**
    A. diameter of the catheter.
    B. viscosity of the fluid.
    C. density of the fluid.
    D. length of the tubing.
    E. system compliance.

84. **Regarding the arterial pressure waveform:**
    A. the fundamental frequency is equal to the heart rate.
    B. the transducer is connected to a Wheatstone bridge.
    C. the flushing device is pressurized to 100 mmHg.
    D. the arterial cannula should be tapered.
    E. the dicrotic notch is related to aortic valve closure.

85. **The following are true with regard to spinal needles:**
    A. a cutting needle (e.g. Quincke) is less likely to damage the dura than a pencil point needle (e.g. Whitacre).
    B. a pencil point needle (e.g. Whitacre) has a side-hole just proximal to the tip.
    C. a stylet is unnecessary for larger bore needles.
    D. the smaller the bore, the less likely the headache.
    E. a 32-G needle cannot be used for injecting cytotoxic drugs.

83. ACDE

84. ABE

An arterial cannula should have parallel walls and is connected to a diaphragm via a heparinized saline column. Arterial pulsation causes movement of the column, which moves the diaphragm. Diaphragmatic movements are transformed into changes in the resistance and current flow through the wires of a transducer. The transducer is connected to a Wheatstone bridge. Information obtained includes:

> systolic, diastolic and mean pressure
> pulse pressure
> heart rate
> left ventricle contractility assessment (upstroke of waveform)
> respiratory swing
> dicrotic notch (due to closure of the aortic valve).

The fundamental frequency (first harmonic) is the heart rate, and the natural frequency is the frequency at which the monitoring system itself resonates and amplifies the signal, and should be at least 10 times the fundamental frequency. It is related as follows:

$$\text{natural frequency} \propto \frac{\text{catheter diameter}}{\sqrt{\text{system compliance} \times \text{length of tubing} \times \text{fluid density}}}$$

85. BD

Spinal needles are either pencil point (e.g. Whitacre and Sprotte) or cutting (e.g. Quincke and Yale). The cutting spinal needles cut the dural fibres and may cause a worse headache due to leakage of cerebrospinal fluid (CSF), whereas the pencil point needles separate the dural fibres and are less traumatic. All the spinal needles should be used with a stylet, whatever the size, to eliminate coring the tissue, and the smaller the needle used the less likelihood there is of developing a dural headache, although the disadvantage of the smaller needles is that CSF drainage is much slower to appear in the hub, and the flexibility of the needle makes the use of introducers necessary, which may themselves pierce the dura.

86. **A pneumotachograph:**
    A. measures gas volume.
    B. relies on turbulent gas flow.
    C. incorporates a heating coil.
    D. detects a pressure change across a fixed resistance.
    E. detects unidirectional gas flow only.

87. **The Bourdon pressure gauge:**
    A. is colour coded for each particular gas or vapour.
    B. does not need to be calibrated.
    C. contains a coiled tube which uncoils when the pressure increases.
    D. measures pressure in proportion to the volume remaining in the case of nitrous oxide.
    E. can cause gases to escape from the back of the casing if the tube ruptures.

88. **Oxygen concentrators:**
    A. extract oxygen from water.
    B. contain aluminium silicates.
    C. contain a molecular sieve that retains argon.
    D. discharge unwanted components to the atmosphere.
    E. deliver a maximum concentration of oxygen of 79%.

89. **The following are true regarding face masks and catheter mounts:**
    A. the Rendell–Baker face mask has an air-filled cuff.
    B. catheter mounts increase deadspace by up to 25 ml.
    C. catheter mounts have 22-mm connections to the breathing system.
    D. excessive face mask pressure may lead to oculomotor nerve damage.
    E. adult face mask deadspace is 10 ml.

86. CD

A pneumotachograph measures gas flow and consists of a tube with a fixed resistance with two pressure transducers either side of the resistance. Gas flows in a laminar pattern (backwards and forwards) and the flow is summated over time to calculate volume. A heating coil is incorporated to prevent water condensation forming which would encourage turbulent flow.

87. ACDE

A Bourdon pressure gauge is used to measure pressures in cylinders. A coiled oval-shaped tube is exposed to the gas at one end and connected to a needle pointer at the other end which moves across a dial. The pressure of the gas causes the coil to unwind and moves the pointer in an amount proportional to the pressure of the gas. Each pressure gauge is calibrated for the particular gas and is both labelled and colour coded. If the coiled tube ruptures, the gas vents from the back of the casing.

88. BD

Oxygen concentrators extract oxygen from air by exposing it to a zeolite (hydrated aluminium silicates of the alkaline earth metals) column which retains nitrogen and other unwanted components, which are then released into the atmosphere. Argon remains in the finished gas and so the maximum concentration of oxygen available is 95%.

89. C

Face masks consist of an edge, body and mount, and are designed to fit snugly over the mouth and nose. Most face masks for adults have a deadspace of up to 200 ml and an air-filled cuff; however, the Rendell–Baker masks have no cuff and are designed for use in children to reduce the deadspace. Excessive face mask pressure may result in facial or trigeminal nerve damage. Catheter mounts have standard connectors of 15 and 22 mm and may increase deadspace by up to 60 ml.

90. **A paramagnetic analyser:**
    A. measures the partial pressure of oxygen in a sample.
    B. measures the partial pressure of nitrogen in a sample.
    C. measures the partial pressure of nitrous oxide in a sample.
    D. is accurate compared with a fuel cell.
    E. can measure the average of inspired and expired gases only.

90. AD

Oxygen has electrons in two unpaired orbits and is attracted to a magnetic field (i.e. it is paramagnetic). A paramagnetic analyser utilizes the principle that in a magnetic field the oxygen molecules are agitated and this results in a change in pressure proportional to the oxygen concentration, which is then detected by a transducer. Analysers are very accurate, sensitive and have a rapid response time.

Paper 3

1. **The following are true of blood and blood products:**
   A. group O rhesus (Rh)-negative blood is the 'universal donor' blood.
   B. the ABO system is inherited in a Mendelian dominant fashion.
   C. stored whole blood contains added calcium, phosphate and dextrose.
   D. red blood cells are commonly resuspended in a solution containing saline, adenine, glucose and mannitol.
   E. stored blood becomes progressively more alkalotic and hypokalaemic with time.

2. **The pharmacokinetic term 'context-sensitive half-time':**
   A. may be calculated from the terminal half-life of elimination.
   B. is only useful for drugs that are highly plasma protein bound.
   C. is shorter for propofol than for alfentanil.
   D. is independent of length of drug infusion.
   E. can only be measured accurately for a one-compartment model.

1. **ABD**

   Group O Rh-negative blood has no antigens and is therefore suitable as universal donor blood; conversely, group AB Rh-positive blood has no antibodies and is the universal recipient. Whole blood is usually stored in a citrate, phosphate and dextrose solution, but most banked blood is separated into its constituent products and the red cells are resuspended. Packed red blood cells have a haematocrit of approximately 60% because, although they are packed red cells, the preservatives and anticoagulants (sodium chloride 140 mmol/l, adenine 1.5 mmol/l, glucose 50 mmol/l and mannitol 30 mmol/l) result in a reduction in the overall haematocrit. All stored blood has reduced levels of 2,3-diphosphoglycerate (2,3-DPG), causing a shift in the oxygen–haemoglobin dissociation curve to the left, and reduced levels of clotting factors and platelets resulting in clotting defects if infused rapidly. Stored blood becomes progressively more acidotic and hyperkalaemic with time.

2. **C**

   The context-sensitive half-time is the time taken for the drug concentration in the central compartment of a multicompartment model to decline by 50%, following termination of an infusion of that drug. It is a particularly useful measurement when considering how quickly blood (and therefore brain) concentrations of a drug will decline following termination of an infusion. After a short infusion, the central compartment level will fall quickly due to both elimination and redistribution to other compartments. Following longer infusions, the level will fall more slowly because of significant drug transfer from the peripheral compartments back into the central one. The 'context' is the length of infusion and indicates that the half-time is related to length of infusion. Values for propofol are shorter than for alfentanil for all infusion times. The half-time cannot be calculated from the terminal half-life of elimination.

   Hughes, M.A., Glass, P.S., Jacobs, J.R. (1992) Context-sensitive half-time in multicompartment pharmacokinetic models for intravenous anesthetic drugs. *Anesthesiology* **76**, 334–41.

3. **The following statements are correct:**
   A. sevoflurane is more potent than isoflurane.
   B. atracurium is more potent than vecuronium.
   C. flumazenil is an inverse agonist.
   D. efficacy cannot be determined from a logarithmic dose–response curve.
   E. efficacy is determined only by the proportion of receptors occupied.

4. **With regard to drug receptors:**
   A. all drugs exert their pharmacological actions through receptor binding.
   B. ligand-gated channels include the nicotinic cholinergic receptor.
   C. G protein-coupled receptors are common for biological amines and many peptide hormones.
   D. membrane-bound protein kinases act as receptors for some peptide hormones.
   E. drug receptors (as distinct from second messenger 'receptors') are not found intracellularly.

3. **All false**

Potency is determined by the mass of drug required to produce a given clinical effect. When considering equi-analgesic doses of morphine and fentanyl, fentanyl is the more potent because only 100 μg is required to achieve the same effect as 10 mg of morphine. Vecuronium (ED_{95} 0.043 mg/kg) is more potent than atracurium (ED_{95} 0.21 mg/kg). With volatile anaesthetic agents, the agent with the lowest minimum alveolar concentration (MAC) is the most potent (isoflurane 1.1% vs sevoflurane 2.0%). Efficacy is the maximum agonist action that can be exerted at any blood level and varies between drugs, even if all receptors are occupied. Comparison of the logarithmic dose–response curves of two or more drugs will reveal both potency and efficacy. An inverse agonist is a drug that binds to a receptor but causes the opposite clinical effect to the usual endogenous ligand or drug. For example, an inverse agonist at a benzodiazepine receptor would bind to the receptor but cause anxiety; flumazenil does not appear to be an inverse agonist in humans (although a few studies have shown a weak effect) but antagonizes both agonist and inverse agonists at benzodiazepine receptors.

4. **BCD**

A receptor is any cellular macromolecule to which a drug binds to exert its effect. There will be a drug-binding domain on the receptor but the domain is not the receptor itself. Several biological agents are sufficiently lipid soluble to cross the plasma membrane and act on intracellular receptors, e.g. nitric oxide stimulates guanylate cyclase to produce cyclic guanosine monophosphate (cGMP) and thyroid hormones act on soluble DNA-binding proteins that regulate specific gene transcription. Receptors for insulin and atrial natriuretic factor are polypeptides that span the plasma membrane. Drug binding to an extracellular domain causes a conformational change in the cytoplasmic domain, causing the enzyme to become active, catalysing phosphorylation of substrate proteins. The nicotinic cholinergic receptor consists of five subunits and the receptor opens a central transmembrane ion channel when the agonist binds to extracellular domains on both α subunits. Some drugs, such as antacids and ion-exchange resins, do not act via receptors.

5. **With reference to G protein-coupled receptor–effector systems:**
   A. the polypeptide chain receptor crosses the cell membrane five times.
   B. activation of the G protein occurs via the carboxyl-terminal tail of the receptor.
   C. the ligand-binding domain is situated extracellularly.
   D. the system can produce signal amplification.
   E. there is only one form of G protein.

6. **The following are correct examples of isomeric forms:**
   A. tautomer: isoflurane and enflurane.
   B. enantiomer: keto and enol forms of thiopentone.
   C. racemic: *cis*-atracurium.
   D. structural: *S* and *R* forms of ketamine.
   E. geometric: *cis* and *trans* forms.

7. **Aspirin:**
   A. is highly (> 80%) plasma protein bound.
   B. crosses the placenta.
   C. reduces normal body temperature.
   D. is a respiratory stimulant.
   E. in low dosage causes a reduction in serum glucose concentration.

5. **D**

G protein-coupled receptors are serpentine polypeptide chains that cross the cell membrane seven times and are a common receptor. The agonist ligands include most biological amines and many peptide hormones. The ligands appear to bind to a domain in the cell wall enclosed by the transmembrane loops of the receptors. Binding leads to a conformational change in the third intracellular loop that activates one of the members of the G proteins. The activated G protein changes the activity of an enzyme (e.g. adenylate cyclase) or an ion channel. The tail appears only to regulate the receptor–G protein interaction. The series of G proteins are classified by their α subunit.

6. **E**

Isomers are chemicals that share the same molecular formula but have differing molecular structures. Isoflurane and enflurane are examples of structural isomers in which the same atoms are arranged in a different configuration. Enantiomers are optically active isomers of the same chemical that may be differentiated by their effect on polarized light. Although the stereoisomers rotate polarized light, the form of the isomer is notated by its structure (S or R) and not by its effect on polarized light (+ or −), and the S form does not always rotate light to the left (−). Tautomers are dynamic forms of the same basic structure, for example the keto and enol forms of thiopentone. A racemic mixture is one that contains isomeric forms, although not all isomers are biologically active. A recent pronouncement from the American Food and Drug Administration (FDA) suggested that drugs should be presented in the (pure) isomeric form that possesses the desired clinical activity. This may explain the recent increase in the number of isomeric forms produced by the pharmaceutical companies.

7. **ABDE**

Aspirin causes irreversible acetylation of the serine part of the enzyme cyclooxygenase. It is highly plasma protein bound and is antipyretic (although it does not reduce body temperature when it is within the normal range), analgesic and anti-inflammatory. Aspirin is a respiratory stimulant and has curious effects: in low dosage it causes a rise in serum uric acid levels and reduction in serum glucose levels, but in high dose has the opposite effect. Aspirin crosses the placenta and also enters breast milk.

8. **Transfusion of fresh frozen plasma (FFP) may be of use in the treatment of:**
   A. heparin overdose.
   B. haemophilia A.
   C. cholinesterase deficiency.
   D. warfarin overdose.
   E. thrombotic thrombocytopenic purpura.

9. **Adenosine:**
   A. has a half-life of 1 hour.
   B. is useful in second-degree heart block.
   C. may cause shortness of breath.
   D. may need to be given in higher doses if the patient is taking dipyridamole.
   E. is effective if given orally.

10. **Trimeprazine (Vallergan) syrup possesses the following properties:**
    A. analgesic.
    B. antiemetic.
    C. antihistamine.
    D. anticonvulsant.
    E. anti-5-hydroxytryptamine.

8. **CDE**

    FFP is obtained either by separation of plasma from whole
    blood or by plasmapheresis. In either case the plasma is frozen
    as soon as possible after collection to preserve labile coagula-
    tion factors. It is expensive, carries the risk (albeit remote) of
    infection and needs to be ABO compatible (although not cross-
    matched). It may be stored for up to 1 year, but when thawed
    should be used immediately. FFP is rich in clotting factors and
    antithrombin III and is helpful in the treatment of congenital
    deficiencies of coagulation factors (e.g. that of factor V) when
    there is no specific factor concentrate available. It is valuable in
    patients with thrombotic thrombocytopenic purpura and
    similar syndromes, and it may be used for the reversal of the
    effects of warfarin associated with severe bleeding. The
    treatment of heparin overdose is protamine and the treatment
    of haemophilia A is factor IX concentrates or deamino-8-D-
    arginine vasopressin (DDAVP). One litre of FFP will completely
    replace the clotting factors of an average adult.

9. **C**

    Adenosine is an endogenous purine nucleoside formed from
    ATP or S-adenosylhomocysteine that is used in the treatment of
    supraventricular tachycardia (SVT). It has a very short half-life
    of less than 10 s due to rapid metabolism to inosine and
    adenosine monophosphate (AMP). A bolus of 3 mg is adminis-
    tered rapidly into a large peripheral vein which is then flushed
    with saline and further doses (up to a total of 12 mg) may be
    given. Side-effects include dyspnoea, flushing and chest pain,
    which are all short-lived, except in patients who suffer from
    asthma (who should not receive adenosine). The effects of
    adenosine are antagonized by aminophylline and potentiated
    by dipyridamole.

10. **BC**

    Trimeprazine is a phenothiazine often given to children as an
    oral premedicant in a dose of 2 mg/kg. It is apricot flavoured
    and, in addition to sedation, has antiemetic and antihistamine
    effects, but less α-adrenergic blocking actions than other
    phenothiazines and is relatively short-acting. Trimeprazine also
    has mild anticholinergic and antidopaminergic effects. It is not
    an analgesic and may cause postoperative restlessness if pain is
    present. It can cause convulsions in susceptible patients.

11. **Diclofenac:**
    A. may be safely given in pregnancy.
    B. is contraindicated in acute intermittent porphyria.
    C. may cause confusion in the elderly.
    D. if administered rectally does not cause peptic ulceration.
    E. may exacerbate asthma.

12. **α-Adrenergic agonists cause:**
    A. hypokalaemia.
    B. increased sweating.
    C. peripheral arteriolar vasoconstriction.
    D. increased insulin secretion.
    E. pupillary constriction.

13. **Rocuronium:**
    A. is an aminosteroid.
    B. is more potent than vecuronium.
    C. is metabolized in the liver.
    D. has a vagotonic effect.
    E. has active metabolites.

11. BCE

Like all non-steroidal anti-inflammatory drugs (NSAIDs), diclofenac may exacerbate asthma in susceptible individuals and can still cause peptic ulceration even if administered rectally (by which route it is very effective), although it is classed as intermediate risk (azapropazone is considered high risk and ibuprofen low risk). Like mefenamic acid and piroxicam, diclofenac is contraindicated in porphyria. Diclofenac may impair renal blood flow due to inhibition of renal prostaglandins, and enters synovial fluid a few hours after its peak concentration in the blood. It is more than 99% plasma protein bound and less than 1% is excreted unchanged in the urine. Diclofenac should not be used during pregnancy as it may result in uterine inertia and fetal premature closure of a patent ductus arteriosus, but is often given for analgesia following childbirth.

12. BC

The α-agonists (such as noradrenaline) cause arteriolar smooth muscle constriction, pupillary dilatation, sweating, contraction of the internal urethral sphincter, ejaculation, and reduction in the secretion of insulin, glucagon and antidiuretic hormone (ADH).

13. AC

Rocuronium is an aminosteroid similar in structure to vecuronium and pancuronium. It is less potent than vecuronium, which is an advantage in that, because it is given in a relatively high dose, more molecules arrive at the neuromuscular junction and therefore onset of action is quicker. Rocuronium is administered as an initial dose of 0.6 mg/kg, twice the ED_{95} dose (effective dose that results in 95% twitch reduction from control), and intubating conditions are excellent at 1 min with full paralysis at 2 min and recovery in 30–40 min; repeat bolus doses of 0.15 mg/kg are given. Rocuronium is metabolized in the liver and excreted in bile; 30% is excreted unchanged by the kidney (thus recovery from neuromuscular blockade may be prolonged in patients with renal failure). There are no active metabolites (unlike pancuronium and vecuronium) and infusions may be clinically useful. Rocuronium causes no histamine release and may have some vagolytic action similar to pancuronium, especially if given in a dose of greater than 0.9 mg/kg.

Hunter, J.M. (1996) Rocuronium: the newest aminosteroid neuromuscular blocking drug. *British Journal of Anaesthesia* **76**, 481–3.

14. **The following drugs should be avoided in untreated renal failure:**
    A. pethidine.
    B. atracurium.
    C. enflurane.
    D. diclofenac.
    E. morphine.

15. **The following drugs cause direct renal damage:**
    A. lithium.
    B. cyclosporin A.
    C. hydralazine.
    D. high molecular weight dextrans.
    E. methysergide.

16. **There are theoretical reasons to avoid the following drugs in severely asthmatic patients:**
    A. ketamine.
    B. pancuronium.
    C. morphine.
    D. diclofenac.
    E. neostigmine.

14. ACD

Pethidine is converted to nor-pethidine (a proconvulsant), which may accumulate in renal failure; morphine is metabolized to an active metabolite, morphine-6-glucuronide, that can accumulate but this merely implies that doses of morphine should be titrated to response rather than avoided; alfentanil is currently the safest opioid to use in renal failure. Diclofenac reduces prostaglandin synthesis and thus renal blood flow. With enflurane, 2% of the administered dose is metabolized, resulting in the production of inorganic fluoride ions. Serum levels of fluoride ions are well below the toxic level of 50 µmol/l in normal clinical use, but may increase to dangerous levels if administered for prolonged periods in patients with renal failure. However, the toxic threshold of 50 µmol/l was suggested from studies with methoxyflurane and may not be appropriate for sevoflurane or enflurane because of the lack of tubular metabolism of the latter drugs.

15. ABD

Drugs that cause renal damage may be classified as shown in the table.

Direct acting
Tubular damage, e.g. cyclosporin A, high molecular weight dextrans, aminoglycosides
Nephrogenic diabetes insipidus, e.g lithium
Renal papillary necrosis, e.g. phenacetin
Indirect acting
Allergic, e.g. drug-induced systemic lupus erythematosus (hydralazine, isoniazid, penicillamine)
Retroperitoneal fibrosis, e.g. methysergide

16. CDE

Morphine causes histamine release, all NSAIDs may make asthma worse and neostigmine may cause bronchoconstriction. Ketamine may be actively beneficial in alleviating bronchospasm.

17. **Omeprazole:**
    A. is a proton pump inhibitor.
    B. induces liver enzymes.
    C. is given once a day.
    D. may cause nausea and vomiting.
    E. may cause carcinoid tumours in the stomachs of experimental rats.

18. **The following antibiotics are bacteriostatic rather than bactericidal:**
    A. cephalosporins.
    B. erythromycin.
    C. metronidazole.
    D. tetracyclines.
    E. chloramphenicol.

19. **The following are true with regard to phenytoin:**
    A. chronic administration results in liver enzyme induction.
    B. it has a high therapeutic index.
    C. it is the treatment of choice for petit mal epilepsy.
    D. it may cause cerebellar disorders.
    E. it can result in the development of megaloblastic anaemia.

20. **Methohexitone:**
    A. may cause convulsions.
    B. causes less hypotension than thiopentone.
    C. causes involuntary movements on intravenous injection.
    D. is safer to use than thiopentone in asthmatic patients.
    E. should be avoided in patients suffering from porphyria.

17. **ACDE**
Omeprazole is a proton pump inhibitor (it blocks the H^+/K^+ ATPase enzyme system in the gastric parietal cell), is a liver enzyme inhibitor and has been shown to cause gastric hyperplasia and, rarely, the development of carcinoid tumours in the stomachs of experimental rats. It is used clinically in combination with antibiotics in the treatment of *Helicobacter pylori* infections and the Zollinger–Ellison syndrome. Omeprazole tablets are available in containers with a desiccant, and side-effects include nausea and vomiting, headache, rash and occasionally angioedema.

18. **BDE**

Bactericidal antibiotics	Bacteriostatic antibiotics
Penicillins, cephalosporins, vancomycin	Tetracyclines
Aminoglycosides	Chloramphenicol
Metronidazole	Erythromycin, clindamycin, lincomycin
Rifampicin	
Trimethoprim	

19. **ADE**
Phenytoin has a narrow therapeutic range and serum levels should be monitored. In chronic usage it causes liver enzyme induction but is the first-choice drug for the treatment of grand mal epilepsy (sodium valproate is the first-choice drug for treatment of petit mal epilepsy). Side-effects of phenytoin include the development of megaloblastic anaemia (due to impaired folate metabolism), cerebellar disorders, acne, gum hyperplasia, hirsutism, osteomalacia and teratogenicity.

20. **ABCDE**
Methohexitone is an oxybarbiturate with a pK_a of 7.9 and at pH 7.4 is 25% ionized. Methohexitone can cause muscular twitching and hiccups after injection, although the incidence is reduced by pretreatment with opioids; it may cause convulsions in susceptible individuals. Compared with thiopentone there is less histamine release and cardiovascular depression, but greater respiratory depression, and it should be avoided in patients suffering from porphyria.

21. **Sevoflurane:**
    A. is non-irritant to the airway.
    B. has an MAC value of about 2%.
    C. is less than 2% metabolized.
    D. is contraindicated in patients susceptible to malignant hyperthermia.
    E. compound A, a degradation product formed when sevoflurane circulates through soda lime, is hepatotoxic.

22. **The following drugs are recommended by the European Resuscitation Council in the treatment of supraventricular tachycardia (SVT):**
    A. esmolol.
    B. digoxin.
    C. amiodarone.
    D. sotalol.
    E. adenosine.

21. ABD

Sevoflurane is a recently introduced volatile anaesthetic agent; it is a methyl-isopropyl ether that is non-irritant and useful for inhalational inductions in children as it induces anaesthesia quickly when administered in high concentrations (6–8%). Like all volatile anaesthetic agents it should be avoided in patients susceptible to malignant hyperthermia. The degradation product, Compound A (a vinyl ether), which is produced if sevoflurane circulates through soda lime, has been shown to cause nephrotoxicity (renal tubular damage) in rats exposed to between 50 and 114 parts per million (ppm) after 1 hour of exposure. In human studies the maximum levels recorded have been 32 ppm (well below the predicted toxic range of 150–200 ppm), although there is a theoretical risk of toxicity if very low (less than 1 l/min) fresh gas flows are employed and there is an increase in temperature. For these reasons minimum flow rates of 2 l/min have been recommended when sevoflurane is used in circle systems. (See table in Paper 1, question 14.)

22. ABCE

The European Resuscitation Council have produced the following algorithm for the treatment of SVT:

  initially attempt vagal manoeuvres and then give intravenous adenosine;

  if this does not result in a return to sinus rhythm and there are no adverse signs (such as hypotension or syncope) then try intravenous esmolol, digoxin, verapamil, amiodarone or attempt overdrive cardiac pacing;

  if there are adverse signs, immediately perform synchronized DC shock, then give a loading dose of intravenous amiodarone and repeat DC shocks until successful restoration of sinus rhythm.

23. **Claims that ropivacaine is superior to bupivacaine include the fact(s) that ropivacaine is:**
    A. more potent.
    B. shorter in onset of action.
    C. longer acting.
    D. less likely to cause motor blockade.
    E. less cardiotoxic in overdose.

24. **The following are mixtures of isomers:**
    A. atracurium.
    B. mivacurium.
    C. bupivacaine.
    D. ropivacaine.
    E. ibuprofen.

25. **Aminophylline:**
    A. is a mixture of theophylline and ethylenediamine.
    B. is metabolized by xanthine oxidase.
    C. has an elimination half-life of 12 hours.
    D. causes peripheral vasodilatation.
    E. is a central nervous system (CNS) stimulant.

23. DE

Ropivacaine is a new long-acting single isomer local anaesthetic of the amide type. It has a molecular weight of 274 daltons, is 94% plasma protein bound and has a pKa of 8.1. Most studies have shown a similar onset, duration and offset time for sensory blockade as compared with a similar dose of bupivacaine, but its stated advantages over bupivacaine include less motor blockade and reduced likelihood of cardiovascular toxicity if accidentally administered intravascularly.

McClure, J.H. (1996) Ropivacaine. *British Journal of Anaesthesia* **76**, 300–7.

24. ABCE

Drugs that have an asymmetric centre or plane of symmetry within their molecular structure are said to be chiral. They are available as pairs of non-superimposable mirror images called enantiomers that share essentially the same physicochemical properties. These three-dimensional structural differences can translate into enantio-specific pharmacological or pharmaco-kinetic properties that may be important in understanding the clinical pharmacology of chiral drugs. Many chiral drugs are available as the racemate in which equal proportions of the two enantiomers are administered concurrently. In the above, ropivacaine is the only single isomer.

25. ABDE

Aminophylline is a bronchodilator; the ethylenediamine component is added to make theophylline water soluble. Aminophylline is a positive inotrope and chronotrope, and a peripheral vasodilator. It induces diuresis (by reducing renal tubular reabsorption) and stimulates gastric secretions. There is CNS stimulation, which not only increases respiration but may precipitate convulsions. Aminophylline is metabolized in the liver by xanthine oxidase and has a half-life of approximately 5 hours, although this is decreased in cigarette smokers and increased if patients are taking enzyme inhibitors such as cimetidine.

26. **Sodium nitroprusside (SNP):**
    A. is degradable by sunlight.
    B. may cause methaemoglobinaemia.
    C. overdose is treated with hydroxocobalamin.
    D. may cause lactic acidosis.
    E. toxicity is confirmed by measuring serum or urine thiocyanate levels.

27. **Propranolol:**
    A. is a non-selective β-adrenergic antagonist.
    B. has intrinsic sympathomimetic activity (ISA).
    C. crosses the blood–brain barrier.
    D. has an active metabolite.
    E. has local anaesthetic activity.

26. ABCDE

SNP is a directly acting vasodilator that is administered intravenously in a dose of 0–10 µg/kg per min (maximum total dose 1.5 mg/kg). SNP is photodegradable and turns blue if exposed to sunlight and thus has to be protected by silver foil. It causes arteriolar and venous dilatation and may reduce arterial oxygen tension due to pulmonary artery vasodilatation (effectively increasing ventilation–perfusion mismatch). There is reflex tachycardia during use and a rebound increase in blood pressure on discontinuation of the drug. SNP is metabolized by liver rhodenase but, if given in excessive amounts, enters red blood cells and is converted to methaemoglobin and an unstable nitroprusside radical. This may be converted to a cyanide radical which inhibits cytochrome oxidase (responsible for oxidative processes), resulting in anaerobic metabolism and the development of lactic acidosis. The unstable nitroprusside radical is ultimately transformed to thiocyanate (excessive amounts are neurotoxic), which can be measured in the urine or plasma. Treatment of toxicity is with hydroxocobalamin, which is transformed to cyanocobalamin, a less toxic compound than the nitroprusside radical.

27. ACDE

Propranolol is a non-selective β-adrenergic blocker with local anaesthetic properties (in high dosage) but no intrinsic sympathomimetic activity. It is almost completely absorbed after oral administration, but one-third of the administered dose is metabolized on first passage through the liver. Propranolol is 90–95% plasma protein bound and lipid soluble (therefore it crosses the blood–brain barrier and may cause nightmares as a side-effect). There is one active metabolite that possesses clinical activity. Like other β blockers propranolol may precipitate bronchospasm in asthmatic patients and can mask the signs of hypoglycaemia in diabetic patients.

28. **The following drugs should be avoided in patients currently taking monoamine oxidase inhibitors (MAOIs):**
    A. pethidine.
    B. morphine.
    C. fentanyl.
    D. ephedrine.
    E. bupivacaine.

29. **Bupivacaine:**
    A. is an aromatic amine with an ester link.
    B. is bound to α_1-acid glycoprotein.
    C. crosses the placenta in clinically significant amounts.
    D. is given in a maximum single dose of 3 mg/kg.
    E. in toxic doses may prolong the Q–T interval on the ECG.

30. **Ondansetron:**
    A. is a dopamine antagonist.
    B. is better at controlling nausea than emesis.
    C. causes sedation.
    D. is expensive relative to metoclopramide.
    E. is not licensed for use in children under the age of 10.

28. ACD

The number of prescriptions written for MAOIs has decreased in recent years due to the development of improved drugs for the treatment of depression, but occasionally one meets a patient taking MAOIs. Ideally, MAOIs should be discontinued 2 weeks before surgery as their main effect is to increase the stores of catecholamines. The actions of indirectly acting drugs such as ephedrine are potentiated and the following may interact, producing clinical effects similar to those of a phaeochromocytoma:

tyramine-containing foods such as cheese, Marmite, Bovril and red wine
pethidine, fentanyl and alfentanil
tricyclic antidepressants.

Morphine is the safest opioid to use and although local anaesthetics are safe, ephedrine must be avoided.

29. BE

Bupivacaine is an aromatic amine with an amide link. It is a weak base with a pK_a of 8.1 and is bound to α_1-acid glycoprotein; it crosses the placenta in small amounts (only 5% is unbound, of which 15% is unionized and therefore a total of only 0.75% of administered dose crosses the placenta). In the UK the maximum recommended dose is 2 mg/kg per 4-hour period. With accidental intravascular injection precipitous hypotension, cardiac dysrhythmias and atrioventricular block may occur. Slow dissociation from the sodium channel binding sites is responsible for the prolonged cardiac toxicity. Treatment with bretylium specifically reverses bupivacaine-induced cardiac depression.

30. BD

Ondansetron is a $5HT_3$ (5-hydroxytryptamine) antagonist that is relatively expensive and causes a reduction in the incidence of postoperative nausea compared with other antiemetics, but probably not the incidence of vomiting. It is licensed for use in children receiving chemotherapy. It does not cause sedation or oculogyric problems.

31. **The following relate to pulmonary function tests in a 70 kg adult:**
    A. a forced expiratory volume in 1 s (FEV_1)/forced vital capacity (FVC) ratio of 0.9 is consistent with a restrictive lung disorder.
    B. a functional residual capacity (FRC) of 2500 ml is normal.
    C. chronic obstructive pulmonary disease results in decreased total lung capacity (TLC).
    D. a minute volume of 3 l is normal.
    E. FRC is increased under general anaesthesia.

32. **In the immune response to surgery:**
    A. tissue injury results in the release of cytokines.
    B. cytokines mediate non-specific immune responses.
    C. the specific immune response is activated by B lymphocytes.
    D. the immune response can be attenuated by high-dose opioid anaesthesia.
    E. certain subsets of T cell inhibit the immune response.

33. **The following are correct scores in the Glasgow Coma Scale:**
    A. lowest possible score = 0.
    B. opening eyes to command = 2.
    C. flexion of limbs to pain = 3.
    D. verbal confusion = 4.
    E. unilateral fixed dilated pupil = 2.

34. **Dietary lack of essential fatty acids results in:**
    A. oily skin.
    B. hirsutism.
    C. reduced platelet numbers.
    D. impaired wound healing.
    E. hypoglycaemia.

31. AB

An FEV_1/FVC ratio of 0.9 may be present in patients with normal lungs or in patients with a restrictive lung disease; in the latter, however, the lung volumes are reduced proportionally. Patients with chronic obstructive pulmonary disease have a reduced FVC but an increased residual volume and FRC, resulting in an increased TLC. The normal minute volume is approximately 70–100 ml/kg body weight and so should be approximately 5.7 L in the example above. FRC is reduced when supine and is further reduced during general anaesthesia.

32. ABCDE

A comprehensive review of this subject can be found in the reference below. Both high-dose opioid anaesthesia and regional blockade can be used to attenuate the immune response to surgery, though whether this is desirable or not has yet to be elucidated.

Sheeran, P., Hall, G.M. (1997) Cytokines in anaesthesia. *British Journal of Anaesthesia* **78**, 201–19.

33. CD

Glasgow Coma Scale (GCS)		
Best verbal response	**Best eye opening**	**Best motor response**
None = 1	None = 1	None = 1
Incomprehensible = 2	To pain = 2	Extends to pain = 2
Inappropriate = 3	To voice = 3	Flexes to pain = 3
Confused = 4	Spontaneous = 4	Withdraws to pain = 4
Orientated = 5		Localizes to pain = 5
		Normal = 6

Lowest possible score = 3
Highest possible score = 15
Coma is defined as a GCS of less than 8

34. CD

A normal diet should contain approximately 50% of the fat content as essential fatty acids (linoleic and linolenic acids). Lack of these essential fatty acids results in dry skin, alopecia, hepatomegaly, thrombocytopenia and impaired wound healing.

35. Deviation of the trachea to the right occurs in:
  A. right-sided tension pneumothorax.
  B. massive left empyema.
  C. right upper lobe collapse.
  D. right-sided bronchiectasis.
  E. right pneumonectomy.

36. Features of hyperthyroidism include:
  A. pretibial myxoedema.
  B. finger clubbing.
  C. weakness of the thigh muscles.
  D. cerebellar dysfunction.
  E. anaemia.

37. Primary hyperaldosteronism (Conn's syndrome) is associated with the following:
  A. hypokalaemia.
  B. increased serum renin levels.
  C. adrenal cortical hyperplasia in approximately half the cases.
  D. renal artery stenosis.
  E. increase in urinary sodium excretion.

38. Addisonian crisis is associated with:
  A. hypokalaemia.
  B. increased serum renin levels.
  C. hypertension.
  D. fever.
  E. hypoglycaemia.

35. BCE
Deviation of the trachea to the right will occur in the following conditions: left-sided tension pneumothorax, empyema or haemothorax; right-sided lung collapse or pneumonectomy.

36. ABC
Clinical features of hyperthyroidism include:

thyroid gland: smooth enlargement +/ − bruit
eye: exophthalmos, lid lag, chemosis, proptosis, lid retraction
cardiovascular: tachycardia or atrial fibrillation
gastrointestinal: weight loss and diarrhoea despite a good appetite
skin: palmar erythema, clubbing of the fingers, excessive sweating, warmth intolerance and pretibial myxoedema
others: difficulty with sleeping, proximal myopathy and resting tremor.

37. AC
Conn's syndrome is due to either adrenal cortical hyperplasia (50%) or a benign adrenal adenoma (50%). Increased aldosterone levels cause sodium retention and hypertension as well as reduced potassium levels. Serum renin levels are reduced and treatment is with spironolactone or surgery. Secondary hyperaldosteronism may be due to renal artery stenosis, congestive cardiac failure, nephrotic syndrome or cirrhosis. These conditions cause an increase in serum renin levels and peripheral oedema.

38. DE
Addisonian crisis (acute symptomatic hypoadrenalism) usually occurs in patients taking steroids who have suddenly stopped taking the drug or are exposed to stress (such as surgery). It is associated with fever, hyponatraemia, hyperkalaemia, hypotension, hypoglycaemia, ST segment depression on the ECG and a raised erythrocyte sedimentation rate (ESR). Treatment is by maintenance of circulating volume and immediate intravenous steroid replacement.

39. **Sudden onset of complete heart block is associated with:**
    A. an increase in stroke volume.
    B. reduced exercise tolerance.
    C. variable loudness of the first heart sound.
    D. absent *a* waves in the central venous pressure waveform.
    E. syncope.

40. **Bradykinin:**
    A. is a peptide.
    B. causes smooth muscle dilatation.
    C. increases capillary permeability.
    D. production is reduced by the administration of aprotinin.
    E. is metabolized by angiotensin-converting enzyme (ACE).

41. **The following substances cause the release of the linked hormone from the anterior pituitary:**
    A. somatostatin – growth hormone.
    B. dopamine – prolactin.
    C. luteinizing hormone releasing hormone (LHRH) – follicle stimulating hormone (FSH).
    D. progesterone – luteinizing hormone (LH).
    E. thyroxine – thyroid stimulating hormone (TSH).

42. **The QRS deflection on the ECG:**
    A. is normally longer than 0.2s.
    B. is associated with ventricular repolarization.
    C. is abnormally prolonged in bundle branch block.
    D. is associated with the phase of isovolumetric ventricular contraction.
    E. is absent in complete heart block.

39. **ABCE**

The onset of complete heart block is associated with an increase in the stroke volume due to ventricular bradycardia and increased diastolic time, varying loudness of the first heart sound (due to closure of the atrioventricular valves, which may coincide with ventricular contraction) and syncope. Absent *a* waves in the central venous pressure waveform occur in atrial fibrillation; however, cannon waves may be seen in complete heart block due to atrial contraction against a closed atrioventricular valve.

40. **ACDE**

Bradykinin is a peptide consisting of nine amino acids produced from the breakdown of high molecular weight kininogen by plasma kallikrein. It increases capillary permeability, causes smooth muscle contraction and encourages chemotaxis (like the effects of histamine). Bradykinin is broken down by ACE and its production is reduced in the presence of aprotinin (a kallikrein inhibitor).

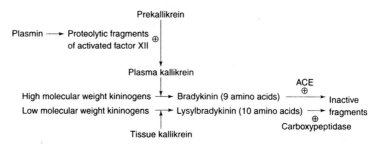

41. **C**

Somatostatin reduces growth hormone release. Dopamine (prolactin inhibiting factor) reduces prolactin release. Progesterone and thyroxine both inhibit release by negative feedback.

42. **CD**

The QRS deflection represents ventricular depolarization and is normally less than 0.12 s in duration. It is still present in complete heart block, although independent of the P wave. Abnormal prolongation of the QRS complex occurs in bundle branch block, ventricular ectopic beats, ventricular hypertrophy, hyperkalaemia and Wolff–Parkinson–White syndrome.

43. Physiological changes in the elderly include:
  A. increase in serum creatinine concentration.
  B. increase in pain threshold.
  C. increase in chest wall compliance.
  D. reduction in basal metabolic rate.
  E. reduced volume of the epidural space.

44. Sensory loss occurs in:
  A. bulbar palsy.
  B. tabes dorsalis.
  C. carpal tunnel syndrome.
  D. poliomyelitis.
  E. syringomyelia.

43. **BDE**

It is normal for the urea concentration to increase in elderly patients, but serum creatinine should remain within the normal range because the reduction in excretion is compensated for by the reduction in production due to reduced muscle mass. Changes in the elderly include those shown in the table.

Cardiovascular

Increased incidence of hypertension and ischaemic heart disease and reduction in cardiac output

Respiratory

Reduction in vital capacity, lung and chest wall compliance, impaired response to hypoxia and hypercarbia and an increase in FRC and the tendency of small airways to collapse

Others

Reduction in cerebral, renal and liver blood flow

Increase in the proportion of body fat

Increase in cerebrospinal fluid (CSF) pressure and reduction in the volume of the epidural space

Sensitivity to CNS depressants

Increase in pain threshold

Reduction in basal metabolic rate

---

44. **BCE**

Bulbar palsy and poliomyelitis are pure motor illnesses with no sensory involvement. Tabes dorsalis is due to syphilis and affects the spinal cord dorsal columns (vibration and positional senses especially), whilst carpal tunnel syndrome is due to median nerve entrapment. In syringomyelia the first signs are a dissociated cutaneous sensory loss (loss of pain and temperature with preservation of light touch) in the upper limbs associated with loss of reflexes.

45. **Poorly controlled diabetes mellitus in pregnancy may result in the following:**
    A. oligohydramnios.
    B. a larger than normal baby.
    C. fetal spinal abnormalities.
    D. pre-eclamptic toxaemia.
    E. hypoglycaemia in the neonate.

46. **Sickle cell trait is associated with the following:**
    A. anaemia.
    B. positive Sickledex test.
    C. the condition is more common in caucasians than Afro-Caribbeans.
    D. preoperative exchange transfusion may be required for all but the most minor procedures.
    E. blood cells will sickle if the arterial oxygen saturation drops to 90%.

47. **The residual volume in the lung is increased in the following conditions:**
    A. phrenic nerve palsy.
    B. an acute attack of asthma.
    C. bronchiectasis.
    D. emphysema.
    E. pulmonary embolus.

45. **BCDE**

Poorly controlled diabetes in the pregnant woman may affect the pregnancy in the following ways:

> in the mother: polyhydramnios, pre-eclamptic toxaemia (increasing the risk of death in the mother 10-fold) and urinary tract infections;
>
> in the fetus: macrosomia (large baby), increase in intra-uterine death, increase in malformations such as spinal abnormalities and ventriculoseptal defects, infant respiratory distress syndrome and postnatal fetal hypoglycaemia.

Pregnancy may affect diabetic control:

> glycosuria is unreliable and blood sugar levels should be checked regularly;
>
> mothers should be changed to a regular short-acting insulin and needs usually increase during pregnancy;
>
> following delivery of the baby, maternal insulin requirements decrease.

46. **B**

Sickle cell anaemia is a hereditary condition that was an evolutionary development because it provided red blood cell protection against malaria. It usually occurs in people of Afro-Caribbean descent and is due to an amino acid change (valine in place of glycine) in position 6 of the β-haemoglobin chain. Sickle cell anaemia trait is a carrier status and does not cause any symptoms normally; there is a positive Sickledex test (a dye drop test employing sodium metabisulphite) and red blood cells will only sickle at extreme levels of hypoxia (less than the normal partial pressure of oxygen in venous blood). As a general rule the patient should be kept warm, well hydrated, well oxygenated, normotensive and limb tourniquets should be avoided.

47. **BD**

The residual volume is the air left in the lungs after a maximal expiratory effort (about 1 litre in normal adults) and is equal to the FRC minus the expiratory reserve volume (ERV). Residual volume is increased in emphysema and acute asthma.

48. **Secretion of gastric acid is increased by:**
    A. vasoactive intestinal peptide (VIP).
    B. gastrin.
    C. vagal stimulation.
    D. secretin.
    E. somatostatin.

49. **When considering the effects of progressive thermal loss from a patient:**
    A. hypothermia is defined as a core temperature of less than 35°C.
    B. the oxygen–haemoglobin dissociation curve is shifted to the left.
    C. consciousness is lost at 30°C.
    D. U waves appear on the ECG.
    E. Electroencephalography (EEG) activity ceases at 25°C.

48. **BC**

Hydrochloric acid is secreted by the parietal cells of the stomach body. Parietal cells contain small channels (canaliculi) that communicate with the lumens of the gastric glands. Gastric acid kills ingested bacteria, aids protein digestion and stimulates the flow of bile and pancreatic juice. The table shows the factors that alter the secretion of gastric acid.

Increase	Decrease
Gastrin	VIP
Motilin	Serotonin (5HT)
Vagal stimulation	Gastric inhibitory peptide (GIP)
Histamine H_2 stimulation	Secretin
	Somatostatin

49. **ABC**

Hypothermia is defined as a core temperature below 35°C. It may be caused by immersion in cold water, exposure to the elements, anaesthesia, head injury, alcohol, hypopituitarism, hypoglycaemia and drugs such as phenothiazines. As the body cools there is a reduction in respiratory rate, heart rate and blood pressure, gases become more soluble in the blood and the oxygen–haemoglobin dissociation curve is shifted to the left. Characteristic J waves appear on the ECG and the Q–T interval becomes prolonged. Below 33°C the muscles become rigid and at 30°C there is loss of consciousness. At this temperature basal metabolic rate and cerebral blood flow are 75% of normal and the EEG shows burst suppression. The heart usually deteriorates into ventricular fibrillation below 25°C and there is no EEG activity below 21°C.

50. **Regarding blood pressure control:**
    A. baroreceptors are situated in the carotid body.
    B. baroreceptors in the aortic arch synapse in the nucleus of the tractus solitarius.
    C. baroreceptors have some effect on the respiratory centre.
    D. the vasomotor centre is situated in the medulla.
    E. baroreceptors are stretch receptors located in the adventitial layer of blood vessels.

51. **The exocrine part of the pancreatic gland secretes:**
    A. lipase.
    B. renin.
    C. trypsin.
    D. amylase.
    E. esterase.

52. **The following are true with regard to the microcirculation:**
    A. capillaries have walls composed of a single layer of cells.
    B. arterioles have relatively little muscle.
    C. capillaries have no innervation.
    D. capillary gaps are 5–9 µm wide.
    E. the precapillary sphincters are innervated.

50.   BCDE

Baroreceptors are located in the aortic arch and carotid sinus and the vasomotor centre is situated in the ventrolateral medulla.

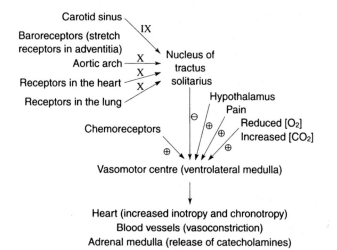

51.   ACDE

The exocrine part of the pancreas consists of glands that resemble salivary glands and secrete zymogen granules discharged into the duct lumen by exocytosis. The ducts combine to form the pancreatic duct (of Wirsung), which joins the common bile duct to form the ampulla of Vater. Pancreatic juice is alkaline and, as well as digestive enzymes, contains sodium, potassium, chloride, magnesium, bicarbonate and sulphate. Secretin causes the release of pancreatic juice that is very alkaline (due to high quantities of bicarbonate) but poor in enzymes, whilst cholecystokinin (CCK) and vagal stimulation cause secretion of pancreatic juice rich in lipase, amylase, trypsin, chymotrypsin, phospholipase A, carboxypeptidases A and B, esterase and elastase.

52.   ACD

Arterioles have a relatively large proportion of muscle and the precapillary sphincters are not innervated but respond to local or circulating substances. When the capillaries are fully dilated red blood cells are able to go through in 'single file'. Capillaries are single layers of cells with gaps and contain 5% of the blood volume at any one time.

53. **The following are true regarding renal blood flow:**
    A. the kidneys receive approximately 20% of the cardiac output.
    B. blood flow to the medulla is high relative to the cortex.
    C. 5HT (serotonin) causes renal vasodilatation.
    D. ADH (vasopressin) causes renal vasoconstriction.
    E. renal blood flow may be estimated using inulin.

54. **Blood buffers include:**
    A. bicarbonate.
    B. haemoglobin.
    C. proteins.
    D. phosphate.
    E. chloride.

53. AD

The kidneys receive 20% of cardiac output, but only consume approximately 8% of total body oxygen consumption. There is differential blood flow within the kidney, with the cortex receiving approximately five times the amount of blood (weight for weight) than the medulla. The factors listed in the table affect renal blood flow.

Vasoconstriction	Vasodilatation
(α_1-Adrenergic receptors)	(Dopamine receptors)
Angiotensin	Dopamine
ADH (vasopressin)	Prostacyclin
5HT (serotonin)	Protein load
Exercise	Pyrogens
Hypoxia	Parasympathetic stimulation

Renal blood flow may be measured using the Fick principle; *p*-aminohippuric acid (PAH) is used because it is filtered, secreted into the proximal convoluted tubule and completely cleared from the plasma. Inulin is used to estimate glomerular filtration rate (GFR).

54. ABCD

Intracellular and extracellular pH are generally maintained at very constant levels by the buffering capacity of the body fluids. A buffer is a substance that has the ability to bind or release hydrogen ions in solution, thus keeping the pH of the solution relatively constant despite the addition of considerable quantities of acid or base. The general equation for a buffer system is:

$$HA \longrightarrow H^+ + A^-$$

where HA is the undissociated acid, H^+ the hydrogen ion and A^- the anion. Blood buffers include: bicarbonate (65%), haemoglobin (29%), proteins (5%) and phosphate (1%).

55. **The following conditions should be excluded as a cause of electromechanical dissociation (EMD):**
    A. disconnection of the ECG leads.
    B. primary brain injury.
    C. hypothermia.
    D. pulmonary embolus.
    E. cardiac tamponade.

56. **The following are true regarding phosphate:**
    A. absorption is increased by the presence of growth hormone.
    B. most of the body phosphate is stored in bone.
    C. increased levels may be seen in patients with acromegaly.
    D. urinary excretion of phosphate is increased by the presence of active Vitamin D.
    E. urinary excretion of phosphate is increased by calcitonin.

55.   CDE

EMD is one of the three types of cardiac arrest (the other two being ventricular fibrillation and asystole). It is defined as the presence of electrical activity on the ECG but with no palpable central pulse and is due to profound myocardial pump failure despite normal or near-normal electrical excitation. It may be caused by any of the factors listed in the table.

Primary (failure of excitation–contraction coupling)
Inferior myocardial infarction
Drugs (β-adrenergic blockers, calcium antagonists, toxins)
Electrolyte abnormalities (hyperkalaemia, hypocalcaemia)
Hypothermia
Secondary (mechanical embarrassment to cardiac output)
Large pulmonary embolus
Tension pneumothorax
Hypovolaemia
Cardiac tamponade
Cardiac rupture
Prosthetic heart valve occlusion
Atrial myxoma or thrombus

Resuscitation comprises life support plus specific treatment if the cause is known or suspected (e.g. calcium in hyper-kalaemia) and adrenaline 1 mg intravenously.

European Resuscitation Council Working Party (1993) Adult advanced cardiac life support: the European Resuscitation Council guidelines. *BMJ* **306**, 1589–93.

56.   ABCE

Phosphate is mainly intracellular, is a component of enzymes (such as ATP) and 2,3-DPG, and is a blood buffer. The usual intake is approximately 35 mmol per day and absorption is increased by the presence of growth hormone. Reductions in serum levels (which may be a cause of tetany) are due to malabsorption, inadequate intake, e.g. in total parenteral nutrition, primary hyperparathyroidism or renal tubular acidosis. Increased levels may be seen in patients with acromegaly or hypoparathyroidism.

57. **Excessive secretion of prolactin:**
    A. is most commonly due to a pituitary tumour.
    B. may occur secondary to hypothyroidism.
    C. causes menorrhagia in females.
    D. results in aggressive sexual behaviour in males.
    E. may result from the use of dopamine antagonists.

58. **The following are true of haemoglobin SC disease:**
    A. it is commonest in eastern Mediterranean people.
    B. patients have a normal haemoglobin level.
    C. it causes a positive Sickledex test.
    D. there are usually target cells visible on the blood film.
    E. the disease may present as a retinal thrombosis.

59. **The following diffuse freely across the placenta:**
    A. IgG.
    B. calcium.
    C. iodine.
    D. glucose.
    E. fats.

60. **The endocrine part of the pancreas secretes:**
    A. glucagon.
    B. VIP.
    C. somatostatin.
    D. 5HT (serotonin).
    E. insulin.

57. ABE

Excessive secretion of prolactin may be due to:

chromophobe adenoma of the anterior pituitary gland (the most common cause)
hypothyroidism
following pregnancy
antidopaminergic agents, such as chlorpromazine
ectopic secretion of prolactin by a carcinoma (usually of the lung).

In females, hyperprolactinaemia causes amenorrhoea and galactorrhoea, whilst in males it results in impotence and galactorrhoea.

58. CDE

Haemoglobin SC disease is a mixture of sickle cell anaemia and haemoglobin C disease and is most common in people of Afro-Caribbean descent. As well as a positive Sickledex test, a blood film will reveal sickle cells and target cells. Patients usually have mild anaemia, haematuria and are at risk of thrombosis and avascular necrosis of bones. Anaesthetic management is similar to that for patients with sickle cell disease.

59. AE

Water, amino acids, fats, IgG and small unionized water-soluble drugs diffuse freely across the placenta. Glucose crosses by facilitated diffusion, whilst calcium and iodine cross by active transport.

60. ACE

The islets of Langerhans are collections of cells present throughout the pancreas (especially the tail) and represent approximately 1–2% of the total gland. They have a copious blood supply that drains into the hepatic portal vein. The majority of the cells are B cells (about 60–75%), which are usually situated in the centre of each islet and are surrounded by the A cells (about 20%). The remainder are D and F cells and these are scattered throughout the islets. The different cells are identified by their morphology and staining characteristics and secrete the following: A cells, glucagon; B cells, insulin; D cells, somatostatin; and F cells, pancreatic polypeptide.

61. **Regarding diathermy equipment:**
    A. the surgeon is fully responsible for the correct use of diathermy equipment.
    B. unipolar diathermy requires less current and is safer than bipolar diathermy.
    C. diathermy may lead to inhibition of an internal pacemaker.
    D. it is safe to use unipolar diathermy when operating on a testis.
    E. diathermy frequencies are in the region 0.5–1.5 MHz.

62. **The concentration of volatile anaesthetic agent emerging from the outlet of a simple (uncompensated) vaporizer is influenced by the following:**
    A. the saturated vapour pressure (SVP) of the agent.
    B. the 'splitting ratio'.
    C. ambient pressure.
    D. the temperature of the anaesthetic agent.
    E. duration of use.

61. CE

Responsibility for the use of diathermy is equally shared between the surgeon and the anaesthetist. Unipolar diathermy requires greater current as the current must pass through the body to the indifferent electrode ('earthing plate'). Bipolar diathermy current travels a short distance between the two hand-held electrodes and hence less current is required. Diathermy burns occur when there is poor contact between the diathermy plate and the patient, resulting in a high current density at the areas of contact, or if some other part of the patient is in contact with a conducting part of the operating table, this offers an alternative route for current flow. Another danger with unipolar diathermy is infarction of any organ raised on a pedicle as the current density becomes very high along the pedicle. If possible, it is best to avoid diathermy in patients with pacemakers but, if used, bipolar is considerably safer than unipolar diathermy. If unipolar diathermy is absolutely necessary then the plate should be situated so that the current flow from the operating site to the plate avoids the heart and pacemaker system.

62. ABCDE

Vaporizer performance can be affected by:

temperature
fresh gas flow
ambient pressure, although negligible clinical effect
back pressure surges, especially due to minute volume divider ventilators
tilting of the vaporizer
liquid levels within the vaporizer e.g. overfilling
carrier gas composition
presence of stabilizers such as thymol.

63. Anaesthetic suction apparatus:
    A. should have high flow and low displacement.
    B. should generate a negative pressure of 400 mmHg.
    C. must have a reservoir.
    D. efficiency will depend upon the viscosity of the matter being aspirated.
    E. should have as large a collection vessel as possible.

64. Expired respiratory volumes during anaesthesia may be measured by:
    A. spirometry.
    B. ultrasonography.
    C. a Wright respirometer.
    D. anemometry.
    E. rotameters.

65. When checking an anaesthetic machine:
    A. it can be performed safely without an oxygen analyser at the common gas outlet.
    B. checking should begin with pipelines and cylinders disconnected.
    C. the common gas outlet should be obstructed to check for leaks.
    D. vaporizer mounting should be checked.
    E. checking the machine may be delegated to an experienced operating department assistant/practitioner.

63. BCD

The essential components of a medical suction system are a vacuum source, suction tubing and a reservoir or collection device. Efficiency will depend upon:

the displacement of the system
the degree of negative pressure generated
the resistance of the suction apparatus
the viscosity of the material to be aspirated.

If the collecting vessel is very large, the time taken for the vacuum to build up will be proportionally greater. Anaesthetic suction requires high displacement with the generation of at least 400 mmHg negative pressure.

64. AC

Spirometers are calibrated bellows that can measure both expired volumes and flow rates. Ultrasound can be used to measure gas flow by the transit time principle: pulses of ultrasound are transmitted through a gas flow and are detected at a fixed distance away. The time taken will alter proportionately with the gas flow. The Wright respirometer measures expired volumes by the rotation of a vane. Anemometry involves the measurement of gas velocity rather than the actual flow rate. A heated element is cooled by a passing stream of gas and the degree of cooling is proportional to the gas velocity at that point. Rotameters are used to accurately regulate gas flow on the anaesthetic machine. Each rotameter must be specifically calibrated for each particular gas.

65. CD

The latest checklist for the anaesthetic machine does not recommend disconnecting gas pipelines but that a 'tug test' should be performed. It is essential to have an oxygen analyser for checking the machine and before giving an anaesthetic. The machine *must be checked by the anaesthetist* before starting a case. A guide to checking the anaesthetic machine has been produced by the Association of Anaesthetists – you must know it!

Association of Anaesthetists of Great Britain and Ireland (1997) *Checklist for Anaesthetic Apparatus 2.* Association of Anaesthetists of Great Britain and Ireland, London.

66. **The following are true with regard to universal precautions against infection:**
    A. they need only be employed for high-risk cases.
    B. eye protection must be worn.
    C. gloves must be worn when dealing with any body fluid.
    D. needles should be resheathed before disposal.
    E. sputum carries a high risk of transmission of HIV.

67. **The following are true regarding lasers:**
    A. laser is an acronym for light and sound emission of radiation.
    B. laser light is monochromatic, coherent and parallel.
    C. lasers have a wavelength in the infrared spectrum.
    D. carbon dioxide is one type of laser used in clinical practice.
    E. they may cause ignition of plastic endotracheal tubes.

66. BC

Universal precautions are designed to be used in all cases and should be adopted as a routine part of anaesthetic practice. Used needles must not be resheathed nor handed from one person to another. High-risk fluids that transmit HIV include blood, amniotic fluid, pericardial fluid, pleural fluid, synovial fluid, CSF, peritoneal fluid, semen and vaginal secretions. Faeces, nasal secretions, sputum, saliva, urine and vomitus are considered low risk for transmission.

Association of Anaesthetists of Great Britain and Ireland (1992) *HIV and Other Blood-borne Viruses: Guidance for Anaesthetists.* Association of Anaesthetists of Great Britain and Ireland, London.

67. BDE

Laser is an acronym for light amplification by stimulated emission of radiation and is a high-energy monochromatic light. Three types of laser are in clinical use: carbon dioxide (used in ear, nose and throat surgery), argon (used for retinal lesions) and Nd-Yag (used in fibrescopes). The laser can cause skin burns and retinal lesions to personnel, and may cause burning and ignition of plastic endotracheal tubes as well as explosions in the presence of flammable gases.

68. **The following exhibit, or closely approximate to, an exponential function:**
    A. lung emptying with passive expiration.
    B. systemic uptake of volatile anaesthetic agent from the lung.
    C. emptying of an oxygen cylinder at constant gas flow.
    D. zero-order kinetics.
    E. decline in blood levels of an intravenous anaesthetic agent following a bolus dose.

69. **With regard to an exponential function:**
    A. one time constant is the time taken for a quantity to fall to approximately 37% of its initial value.
    B. the time constant is derived from the initial rate of decline.
    C. the half-life is constant.
    D. at the end of two half-lives the quantity remaining is virtually zero.
    E. the rate of decline at any moment is related to the quantity present at that time.

70. **The following questions concern pipeline gases:**
    A. compressed air is available at both 4 and 7 bar pressures.
    B. pipeline nitrous oxide comes from a central storage tank.
    C. pipeline oxygen is delivered at 137 bar.
    D. oxygen piping is coloured black.
    E. quality control of piped medical gases is the responsibility of the anaesthetist.

68. **ABE**

See Question 69.

69. **ABCE**

An exponential function is one where the rate of change of a variable is proportional to the magnitude of that variable. This can be expressed mathematically as: $Q = Q_0\, e^{-t}/CR$, where Q is the quantity (Q_0 at time zero), t is time, and CR is the time constant for the particular exponential function. The time constant is the time taken for the amount or concentration to fall to zero if the initial rate of decline was maintained. In one time constant the quantity remaining will have fallen to 37% of the original amount, after two time constants to 13.5% of the original amount (i.e. 37% of 37%) and after three time constants to 5% of the initial amount or concentration. The time taken for an exponential curve to fall to half of its original value is 0.693 of the time constant; this is known as the 'half-time' or 'half-life'. After two half-lives the quantity remaining is 25% of the original amount. Several biological functions approximate to an exponential, e.g. the volume of gas expired in passive expiration. In pharmacology, the wash-in of drug blood levels with a fixed-rate drug infusion is similar. Zero-order kinetics are where the decline is at a fixed rate and is therefore independent of the quantity present. Complex pharmacokinetics may involve several superimposed exponential functions depending upon the distribution of the drug to different body compartments.

70. **A**

Nitrous oxide is delivered from a central bank of cylinders at a pressure of 4 bar. Oxygen may be obtained from a bank of cylinders, but in large hospitals is more likely to be stored in liquid form in a vacuum insulated evaporator. Oxygen piping is coloured white (delivered at 4 bar) and air piping black. Responsibility for quality control of piped gases lies with the hospital pharmacy. The anaesthetist takes responsibility for the supply of gases between the wall outlet and the patient.

71. **The Cardiff Aldasorber scavenging system:**
   A. is an active scavenging system.
   B. contains soda lime.
   C. absorbs nitrous oxide.
   D. absorbs isoflurane.
   E. releases inhalational agents back into the atmosphere if the scavenging system heats up.

72. **With regard to a standard laryngeal mask airway (LMA):**
   A. size 3 has an internal diameter of 9 mm.
   B. the black line should face the upper lip when correctly positioned.
   C. a single LMA may be reused up to 50 times.
   D. it may safely be used in magnetic resonance imaging (MRI) scanning suites.
   E. a large proportion of patients initially have airway obstruction due to downfolding of the epiglottis.

73. **Regarding automatic non-invasive systemic blood pressure monitors:**
   A. the width of the cuff should equal the diameter of the arm.
   B. they are inaccurate if the patient has atrial fibrillation.
   C. they over-read on a fat arm if the cuff is too tight.
   D. they over-read at very low pressures.
   E. they are inaccurate if the patient has complete heart block.

74. **Regarding nasal cannulae, inspired oxygen concentration is dependent upon:**
   A. tidal volume.
   B. respiratory rate.
   C. proportion of mouth to nose breathing.
   D. oxygen flow rate.
   E. volume of the nasopharynx.

71. **DE**

The Cardiff Aldasorber system was developed to absorb waste anaesthetic gases. It is a passive scavenging system consisting of transfer tubing, a canister and charcoal particles. This system has the following disadvantages:

no absorption of nitrous oxide;
there is release of the anaesthetic vapours if the charcoal particles heat up;
an increase in weight of the particles is the only indication that the canister is exhausted.

72. **ABD**

LMAs have a large internal diameter to reduce the work of breathing, e.g. the size 3 has a 9 mm and the size 4 a 10 mm internal diameter. LMAs can be reused up to 40 times, but have metal self-sealing valves and may distort an MRI image; a version of the standard laryngeal mask with a plastic valve is available for MRI use. Reinforced flexible LMAs are now available that are longer in length but have a reduced internal diameter. Up to 10% of insertions result in airway obstruction, usually due to downfolding of the epiglottis.

73. **BCD**

The width of the blood pressure cuff should be at least 20% greater than the arm diameter. The blood pressure under-reads at very high pressures and over-reads at very low pressures. In atrial fibrillation the strength of the pulse down the arm is variable, thus making the measurement inaccurate; in complete heart block there is a regular pulse down the arm and therefore the measurement is accurate.

74. **ABDE**

Nasal cannulae utilize the venturi effect to entrain air through the nose or mouth and concentration is independent of whether the patient is breathing through the nose or the mouth. They are more comfortable than face masks, although the maximum flow is limited to 4 l/min (which produces an oxygen concentration of 28–30%) as they become uncomfortable at higher oxygen flow rates.

75. With regard to Tuohy needles and epidural catheters:
  A. standard bore is 14G.
  B. standard length is 8 cm.
  C. Huber angle is at 20° to the shaft.
  D. epidural catheter length is 90 cm.
  E. the standard filter is 10 μm.

76. High-frequency jet ventilators:
  A. are time cycled.
  B. provide inspiration for up to 50% of the cycle.
  C. provide an accurate fraction of inspired oxygen (F_{IO_2}).
  D. deliver positive end-expiratory pressure (PEEP) if the respiratory rate is greater than 100 per min.
  E. deliver a minimum minute volume of 20 l/min.

77. The White double-lumen endobronchial tube:
  A. has three cuffs.
  B. has an anterior and lateral curve.
  C. is designed for insertion into the right main bronchus.
  D. has a carinal hook.
  E. has an eye in the bronchial cuff.

78. The emergency oxygen flush:
  A. is usually activated by a non-locking button.
  B. produces a flow rate of 45 l/min.
  C. provides a pressure of 100 kPa.
  D. is arranged so as not to cause barotrauma to the patient.
  E. may dilute anaesthetic gases and cause awareness.

75. CD

The standard Tuohy needle is 16G and 10 cm long (a 15-cm long needle is also available). The Huber angle at the tip is blunt to help prevent dural puncture and Lees lines are the 1-cm graduations on the side of the needle. A standard epidural filter is 0.22 μm, which acts as a viral, bacterial and foreign body filter.

76. ABD

High-frequency jet ventilators are time-cycled ventilators employing a Venturi injector and solenoid valves to deliver gases to the trachea. The frequency and minute volumes can be altered within a range of 20–500 cycles per min and 5–60 l/min respectively. The jet and entrained gases impact on the gases already in the airway and cause them to move forward. The inspiratory time is adjustable from 20 to 50% of the cycle time. Expiration is passive due to recoil of the lungs and chest wall, but PEEP is delivered if the rate is greater than 100 per min, and barotrauma can still occur, especially if there is upper airway obstruction.

77. BCDE

The White double-lumen endobronchial tube is designed for insertion into the right main bronchus, and has the following features: a carinal hook, two cuffs and an eye in the bronchial cuff to ventilate the right upper lobe.

78. ABE

The emergency oxygen flush is usually activated by a non-locking button (to prevent accidental continuous oxygen flush which will dilute anaesthetic gases) and bypasses the flowmeters and vaporizers, delivering a flow rate of 45 l/min at a pressure of 400 kPa, which may cause barotrauma.

79. **The standard laryngeal mask airway (LMA):**
    A. may be lubricated with saline.
    B. may be disinfected by 2% glutaraldehyde.
    C. is more likely to be ignited by laser energy than a standard polyvinyl chloride (PVC) tube.
    D. is recommended for use in 40 patients only.
    E. has a cuff that is not permeable to air.

80. **The standard laryngeal mask airway (LMA):**
    A. is constructed from polypropylene.
    B. has the mask meeting the stem at an angle of 30°.
    C. is ideally lubricated with a silicone lubricant.
    D. may be autoclaved at 146–150°C.
    E. contains no ferromagnetic parts.

81. **Intubating fibrescopes:**
    A. have a working length of 50 cm.
    B. contain no suction channel.
    C. have a nominal external diameter of 6 mm.
    D. have a depth of focus from 0.5 to 5 cm.
    E. have a tip angulation of ± 150°.

82. **The following are true regarding fibreoptic equipment:**
    A. a single glass fibre is approximately 20 μm in diameter.
    B. a single fibre consists of a glass core and surrounding cladding glass.
    C. a standard fibrescope contains 1000 fibres.
    D. the source light is of the same intensity as that emerging from the distal end.
    E. the fibrescope should be disinfected using activated glutaraldehyde.

83. **Hot water bath humidifiers:**
    A. contain a thermostatically controlled heating element.
    B. may transmit bacterial infections.
    C. cannot deliver fully saturated gases to the patient.
    D. must be placed at the same level as the mouth of the patient.
    E. deliver gases at a fixed temperature.

79. AD

80. B

The laryngeal mask airway is constructed from silicone rubber, has a cuff that is permeable to air, nitrous oxide and other gases, and has a ferromagnetic part in the valve. The mask is lubricated with saline or water-based lubricants, not silicone as it may weaken or expand the airway. A single airway can be reused up to 40 times and must be autoclaved at a temperature of 134–138°C; it should not be soaked in glutaraldehyde as this may be absorbed into the mask and transmitted to the patient.

81. D

82. ABE

The intubating fibrescope consists of a flexible cord (nominal 4-mm external diameter and 60-cm length) containing bundles of glass fibres. Each bundle consists of 10 000–15 000 fibres each with a diameter of 5–20 µm which transmit light repeatedly, striking and being reflected from the external cladding layer of glass at a similar angle of incidence until it emerges from the opposite end. The tip deflection is ± 120° and the slope has a suction channel.

83. ABE

Hot water bath humidifiers are used mainly in intensive care units. A container of sterile water is heated by a thermostatically controlled element to the desired temperature and gases are then passed through and delivered to the patient fully saturated with water vapour at 37°C. The temperature of the gases at the patient end are measured with a thermistor, and a feedback mechanism ensures that the correct temperature is maintained in the water bath. The apparatus should be kept below the level of the patient to avoid flooding of the airway with condensed water.

84. **The Manley MP3 ventilator:**
    A. is a minute volume divider.
    B. is driven by a high-pressure oxygen source.
    C. contains a single bellows.
    D. contains three unidirectional valves.
    E. can be used for both spontaneous respiration and intermittent positive-pressure ventilation.

85. **The transoesophageal echocardiograph (TOE):**
    A. is placed at a distance of approximately 20 cm from the teeth in adults.
    B. utilizes ultrasound frequency of approximately 4 MHz.
    C. has a probe that needs to be repositioned frequently.
    D. should not be placed in patients with oesophageal varices.
    E. assesses cardiac output allowing for the patient's height and weight.

86. **With regard to the transoesophageal echocardiograph (TOE):**
    A. the distal oesophagus is parallel with the aorta.
    B. use of diathermy is dangerous.
    C. ventricular wall motion abnormalities can be detected.
    D. assessment of stroke volume is possible.
    E. assessment of afterload can be made.

87. **The Doppler equation, when estimating blood flow using the TOE, contains the following parameters:**
    A. frequency of transmitted ultrasound.
    B. speed of light in body tissue.
    C. speed of sound in body tissue.
    D. blood viscosity.
    E. Doppler frequency shift.

84. **ADE**

The Manley MP3 ventilator is a minute volume divider whereby all the fresh gas flow is delivered to the patient by being divided into tidal volume units. A small bellows receives the fresh gas flow continuously and empties directly into the main bellows after a fixed period of time; when the predetermined tidal volume is achieved, the main bellows empties into the patient.

85. **BCDE**

86. **ACDE**

The transoesophageal Doppler probe is inserted into the mouth and down the oesophagus to a depth of 35–40 cm in adults where the oesophagus is parallel with the descending aorta. The probe has a diameter of 6 mm; it contains a transducer angled at 45° and transmits high-frequency sound waves (4 Mhz). Using TOE, some assessment can be made of:

stroke volume
myocardial function
systemic vascular resistance
volaemic status
wall motion abnormalities.

The probe is safe with diathermy use, but tends to migrate and must be repositioned frequently. It should not be used in patients with oesophageal varices because of the risk of bleeding.

87. **ACE**

The Doppler equation is as follows;

$$\text{flow velocity} = \frac{\text{speed of sound in body tissue} \times \text{Doppler frequency shift}}{\begin{array}{c} 2 \times \text{frequency of transmitted ultrasound} \times \\ \text{cosine of angle between sound beam and blood flow} \end{array}}$$

88. **With regard to the Von Recklinghausen oscillometer:**
    A. it consists of a single cuff.
    B. it contains a control lever and release valve.
    C. pressure oscillations appear on the needle at systolic pressure.
    D. pressure oscillations on the needle are maximal at diastolic pressure.
    E. it is unreliable at low blood pressure.

89. **With regard to oxygen stored in vacuum-insulated evaporators (VIEs):**
    A. oxygen is stored at a pressure of 5–10 atmospheres.
    B. oxygen is stored at a temperature of between −150 and −170°C.
    C. the amount of oxygen remaining is indicated on a pressure gauge.
    D. a safety valve opens at 500 kPa to allow the escape of gas if too much pressure builds up.
    E. the latent heat of vaporization warms the oxygen as it enters the delivery pipeline.

90. **Needle valves control knobs attached to flowmeters:**
    A. are colour coded.
    B. are labelled with the particular gas.
    C. have a body made of gold.
    D. are turned clockwise to increase gas flow.
    E. have a screw thread to allow fine adjustment of gas flow.

88. BC

The Von Recklinghausen oscillometer consists of two cuffs: an upper outer cuff over a lower inner sensing cuff. Air is pumped into both cuffs to exceed systolic pressure and an adjustable leak is set up. When systolic pressure is reached, pulsation is detected under the lower cuff and pressure oscillations are transmitted to a needle on the pressure gauge. At mean pressure, the pulsations are maximal and they cease below diastolic pressure. It is reliable even at low pressures.

89. AB

A VIE consists of liquid oxygen at a pressure of 5–10 atmospheres and temperature of between −150 and −170°C surrounded by a vacuum. The container rests on a weighing balance so that the amount of oxygen remaining can be calculated. A pressure regulator allows gas to enter the pipeline at about 400 kPa and to be warmed in a coil of copper tubing. If there is a pressure build-up, a safety valve opens at 1700 kPa to allow escape of gas.

90. ABE

A needle valve controls the flow of gases through the flowmeters by turning the valve in an anticlockwise direction. The body is made of brass and the needle itself has a thread to allow fine adjustments, whilst the knob is labelled and colour coded for the particular gas.

Paper 4

1. **Mivacurium:**
   A. is more potent than vecuronium.
   B. has a prolonged duration of action in patients with low pseudocholinesterase levels.
   C. has a prolonged duration of action in patients with fulminant liver failure.
   D. has an action which is not terminated by the administration of neostigmine.
   E. must not be administered to pregnant women.

2. **When comparing alfentanil with fentanyl:**
   A. alfentanil has the greater clearance.
   B. alfentanil has the smaller volume of distribution.
   C. a greater fraction of alfentanil is unionized at pH 7.4.
   D. percentage plasma protein binding for the two drugs are equal.
   E. alfentanil is more lipid soluble.

1. **BCE**

   Mivacurium is a short-acting non-depolarizing neuromuscular blocker. It is a mixture of three optical isomers and has a $2 \times ED_{95}$ of 0.14 mg/kg; however a bolus dose of 0.2 mg/kg provides good intubating conditions within 2 min and lasts approximately 20 min. Further boluses of 0.1 mg/kg last 15 min and it may be given as an infusion at a rate of 8–10 μg/kg per min. Because mivacurium is metabolized by plasma pseudo-cholinesterase, its effects are prolonged in patients with low cholinesterase levels including those patients with renal or liver failure. There is spontaneous recovery of neuromuscular function, but neostigmine may be administered in the usual way to speed up recovery by 5–6 min. Mivacurium is not licensed for use in pregnancy due to lack of experimental data.

2. **BC**

   Alfentanil has a shorter terminal half-life of elimination than fentanyl, but this is due to the smaller volume of distribution of alfentanil rather than a greater clearance. The onset of action depends on the lipid solubility and the percentage of unbound drug in plasma. The diffusible fraction is the percentage of drug at pH 7.4 that is both unionized and unbound. Both drugs are weak bases.

	Alfentanil	Fentanyl
V_d steady state (l)	27	224
Clearance (ml/min)	240	1500
Terminal half-life (min)	100	180
pK_a	6.5	8.4
Octanol–water coefficient	128	813
Unionized at pH 7.4 (%)	89	9
Plasma protein binding (%)	91	84
Diffusible fraction (%)	8	1.7

3. **The following drugs have a metabolite that possesses a similar clinical action to the parent compound:**
   A. lignocaine.
   B. pethidine.
   C. pancuronium.
   D. midazolam.
   E. diamorphine.

4. **Which of the following statements are correct?**
   A. morphine acts at μ-opioid receptors.
   B. five subgroups of muscarinic receptor have been identified.
   C. acetylcholine must combine with both α subunits of the nicotinic cholinoceptor to open the ion channel.
   D. two subtypes of γ-aminobutyric acid (GABA) receptor have been identified.
   E. two subtypes of α adrenoceptor have been identified.

5. **Cefuroxime is usually effective against the following pathogens:**
   A. *Staphylococcus aureus.*
   B. *Neisseria gonorrhoeae.*
   C. *Pseudomonas aeruginosa.*
   D. *Streptococcus pneumoniae.*
   E. *Haemophilus influenzae.*

3. BCD

Drug	Metabolite(s)	Activity of parent?
Lignocaine	Monoethylglycinexylidide (MEGX)	No
	Glycinexylidide (GX)	No
Pethidine	Nor-pethidine	Yes (also pro-convulsant)
Pancuronium	3-Hydroxypancuronium	Yes (50%)
	17-Hydroxypancuronium	
Midazolam	α-Hydroxymidazolam	Yes (weak)
Diamorphine	Monoacetylmorphine Morphine	No: diamorphine has no analgesic activity, but is a prodrug

4. ABCDE

Morphine is the prototype μ-receptor agonist. Some studies suggest a subdivision into μ_1 and μ_2; opioid peptides and morphine have similar affinities at μ_1 receptors but morphine has greater selectivity for the low-affinity μ_2. There are five subtypes of muscarinic receptor, M_1–M_5. There is greatest homology between M_1, M_3 and M_5 subtypes which lead to inositol trisphosphate production, and between M_2 and M_4 which inhibit cyclic adenosine monophosphate (cAMP) production. The nicotinic cholinoceptor of the electric eel and vertebrate skeletal muscle is a pentamer consisting of 2α, β, γ and δ subunits. The bulk of the non-membrane-spanning domain is on the extracellular surface. Simultaneous binding of two molecules of acetylcholine to both the α subunits are required to open the channel.

5. ABDE

Cefuroxime is a second-generation cephalosporin normally effective against both Gram-positive and Gram-negative aerobic pathogens, especially *H. influenzae* and *N. gonorrhoeae*. It was developed to be less susceptible to the penicillinases and can be administered intramuscularly as well as intravenously. Cefuroxime may cause allergic reactions in 10% of those patients who are sensitive to penicillin (i.e. there is a 10% incidence of cross-sensitivity). Cefuroxime enters the enterohepatic circulation and is renally excreted.

6. **When considering the anticholinesterases:**
   A. neostigmine and edrophonium bind to the enzyme in a similar manner.
   B. neostigmine has a longer duration of action than pyridostigmine.
   C. physostigmine is not used clinically because it has too short a duration of action.
   D. edrophonium produces less muscarinic side-effects than neostigmine.
   E. the measured volume of distribution of neostigmine is equivalent to the extracellular space.

7. **Tramadol:**
   A. is an opioid.
   B. is more efficacious than codeine phosphate.
   C. possesses serotonin agonist properties.
   D. causes less constipation than morphine.
   E. enhances adrenergic pathways.

6. **D**

   The anticholinesterases in clinical use bind to the enzyme at two possible sites, the anionic and esteratic sites. Edrophonium only binds at the anionic site but both neostigmine and pyridostigmine also form a chemical bond at the esteratic site. Pyridostigmine is longer acting than neostigmine in the usual model used, i.e. antagonism of partial neuromuscular blockade induced by a (continuous) infusion of atracurium. Physostigmine is derived from the Calabar bean and is used as a drug of ordeal because, as a tertiary amine, it crosses the blood–brain barrier. This makes it unsuitable for use in the antagonism of residual neuromuscular blockade. Edrophonium has a more rapid onset of action than neostigmine and also produces less unwanted muscarinic side-effects. Although the anticholinesterases are highly ionized, their measured volume of distribution is about three times that of the extracellular space, possibly due to uptake by the liver.

7. **ABCDE**

   Tramadol is an opioid that also possesses serotonin agonist properties and enhances adrenergic pathways. It causes less constipation, addiction potential and respiratory depression compared with morphine, and although it is said to be more efficacious than codeine it is less potent (the usual dose of tramadol being 50–100 mg compared with 30–60 mg codeine). Tramadol may be administered orally or via the intravenous or intramuscular route, but rapid injection may cause convulsions. There is some evidence that tramadol may enhance intra-operative recall during light planes of anaesthesia and adverse psychiatric reactions have been reported with its use. Prolonged elimination of tramadol occurs in renal failure and the dosing interval should be increased in the presence of mild to moderate renal dysfunction; it should be avoided altogether in severe renal failure. Tramadol is not licensed for use in children under the age of 12 or in pregnancy or women who are breast-feeding (tramadol and its metabolites are found in small amounts in human breast milk).

8. **A 4.5% human albumin solution contains:**
   A. clotting factors.
   B. sodium.
   C. preservatives.
   D. protein.
   E. pseudocholinesterase.

9. **Metronidazole:**
   A. is useful against protozoal infections.
   B. may cause epileptiform attacks.
   C. may cause a reaction similar to that of disulfiram (Antabuse) when alcohol is taken simultaneously.
   D. has good oral bioavailability.
   E. may increase the effect of co-administered warfarin.

10. **The following are true regarding dopexamine:**
    A. it causes stimulation of α-adrenergic receptors.
    B. it causes stimulation of dopamine receptors.
    C. it causes stimulation of β_2-adrenergic receptors.
    D. it is useful in the treatment of hypertrophic obstructive cardiomyopathy.
    E. it may be administered safely through a peripheral venous line.

11. **The following may cause extrapyramidal side-effects:**
    A. ketamine.
    B. droperidol.
    C. metoclopramide.
    D. diclofenac.
    E. chlorpromazine.

8. BD

A 4.5% human albumin solution is a heat-inactivated compound derived from human blood donation. It does not require blood group compatibility tests to be performed before administration and is stored at 2–25°C. Albumin solution contains stabilizers, protein (in a concentration of 45 g/l) and sodium (in a concentration of 136 mmol/l) but no preservatives. The main indications for use are:

burns, trauma and pancreatitis
volume replacement in neonates
protein replacement in hypoproteinaemic conditions and following plasma exchange.

9. ABCDE

Metronidazole is useful in the treatment of anaerobic and protozoal infections, including topical treatment of fungating tumours and rosacea, and is usually given as a dose of 400 mg three times a day orally or 500 mg three times a day intravenously. Metronidazole inhibits the liver metabolism of warfarin as well as phenytoin and lithium, thereby increasing serum levels. Metronidazole itself may cause an Antabuse reaction if taken with alcohol, can induce convulsions, and causes an unpleasant taste in the mouth and dark-coloured urine.

10. BC

Dopexamine is a synthetic inotropic agent with agonist actions on both β_2-adrenergic and dopamine receptors. It is given by infusion through a central venous line in a dose of 0–6 μg/kg per min. Adverse effects include arrhythmias, tachycardia, nausea and vomiting and tremor. Dopexamine is contra-indicated in the presence of phaeochromocytomas and left ventricular outflow obstruction.

11. BCE

Extrapyramidal side-effects are caused by drugs that have antidopaminergic actions, and these include droperidol, metoclopramide and chlorpromazine.

12. **Tenoxicam:**
    A. is a non-steroidal anti-inflammatory drug (NSAID).
    B. cannot be administered intravenously.
    C. has an elimination half-life of 60–75 hours.
    D. has a low oral bioavailability.
    E. is a useful analgesic for day-case surgery.

13. **Inhaled prostacyclin (PGI₂) would be expected to:**
    A. cause bronchodilatation.
    B. reduce pulmonary artery pressure.
    C. produce no effects on the systemic circulation.
    D. reduce the shunt fraction.
    E. produce potentially toxic metabolites.

14. **The following are true of inhalational anaesthetic agents:**
    A. halothane is a halogenated hydrocarbon.
    B. isoflurane is a structural isomer of enflurane.
    C. sevoflurane is a fluorinated ether.
    D. desflurane is a halogenated hydrocarbon.
    E. enflurane is a fluorinated methylethyl ether.

12. AC

Tenoxicam is a thenothiazine derivative of the oxicam class of NSAIDs with an oral bioavailability of 99%. It has a long half-life of elimination (thus is administered once daily) and is highly ionized at pH 7.4. It may be given intravenously, which lends itself to perioperative use, and it might therefore be compared with ketorolac (the other NSAID that can be administered intravenously). However, tenoxicam does not appear to be efficacious in day surgery: one study found a single 20 mg i.v. dose to be indistinguishable from placebo in providing analgesia after day-case laparoscopy; in another study tenoxicam 20 mg i.v. provided poorer analgesia compared with diclofenac 75 mg i.m. in the first 3 hours following dental surgery. Tenoxicam is not recommended for use in children, and in common with other NSAIDs is contraindicated in asthma, bleeding diatheses and peptic ulceration.

13. B

Inhaled prostacyclin has been evaluated as a selective pulmonary arterial vasodilator. Since no agent has been found that selectively dilates pulmonary rather than systemic vasculature, selectivity has been attempted by using ultra-short-acting agents applied directly to the pulmonary circulation. Prostacyclin causes vasodilatation in the pulmonary circulation; however its half-life is 2–3 min (compared with only a few seconds for nitric oxide) and high doses cause systemic effects. Prostacyclin may cause bronchoconstriction and certainly does not cause bronchodilatation. Its metabolites do not exert pharmacological actions.

14. ABCE

Isoflurane, enflurane and desflurane are all fluorinated methylethyl ethers. Sevoflurane is a fluorinated ether and halothane is a halogenated hydrocarbon.

15. **Calcium:**
    A. acts as a second messenger.
    B. is bound by the receptor protein calmodulin.
    C. is a predominantly intracellular ion.
    D. binds to adenylate cyclase and G proteins.
    E. is stored in the endoplasmic reticulum.

16. **Papaveretum (Omnopon):**
    A. contains morphine.
    B. contains codeine.
    C. contains noscapine.
    D. contains papaverine.
    E. may be given orally.

17. **The following are true of antiemetics:**
    A. metoclopramide in high dosage blocks $5HT_3$ (5-hydroxy-tryptamine) receptors.
    B. cyclizine acts directly on the chemoreceptor trigger zone.
    C. prochlorperazine may be administered rectally.
    D. dopamine D_2 receptors are located in the chemoreceptor trigger zone.
    E. metoclopramide is a useful antiemetic for motion sickness.

15. **ABE**

Intracellular calcium is stored in the endoplasmic reticulum and some second messengers act by increasing the intracellular concentration either by increasing calcium entry into the cell (from the highly concentrated interstitial fluid) or by increasing release from the endoplasmic reticulum. A common way to translate a signal to a biological effect inside cells is by way of nucleotide regulatory proteins (G proteins) that bind GTP (guanosine analogue of ATP). One family of G proteins are the heterotrimeric G proteins, which consist of three subunits, α, β and γ; when a ligand binds to a G-coupled receptor, GDP bound to the α subunit is exchanged for GTP and the α subunit separates from the other two units and results in a biological effect. Other calcium-binding proteins include troponin (involved in the contraction of skeletal muscle) and calmodulin, which forms a subunit of phosphorylase kinase thereby increasing the activity of this enzyme and resulting in contraction of smooth muscle.

16. **ABDE**

Papaveretum is now formulated as 7.7 mg Omnopon (containing 253 parts morphine, 20 parts codeine and 23 parts papaverine). Previously it contained noscapine, but this was linked to the development of thalidomide-like abnormalities in children of mothers given the drug during early pregnancy and it is not in the formulation now available. Papaveretum has similar effects to the other opioids, including being antagonized by naloxone, and is available orally mixed with aspirin as Aspav (one tablet contains 500 mg of aspirin, 5 mg of morphine, 0.6 mg of papaverine and 0.52 mg of codeine).

17. **ACD**

Metoclopramide is a dopamine D_2 receptor antagonist acting on the chemoreceptor trigger zone. In high dose (as when used during chemotherapy) it has been shown to antagonize $5HT_3$ receptors. It is of no use in the treatment of travel sickness. The action of the antihistamines, including cyclizine, is predominantly via their anticholinergic effects on the vomiting centre and the labyrinthine pathways.

18. **The following drugs readily cross the blood–brain barrier:**
    A. hyoscine.
    B. glycopyrrolate.
    C. benzylpenicillin.
    D. pancuronium.
    E. physostigmine.

19. **Regarding suspected adverse reactions to drugs:**
    A. any adverse reaction to a new drug should be reported.
    B. drug reactions should be reported using the Committee on Safety of Medicines (CSM) yellow card system.
    C. well-recognized serious drug reactions need not be reported.
    D. suspected adverse drug reactions to trial medications should be reported using the CSM yellow card system.
    E. all patients with adverse reactions should receive skin-prick testing.

20. **The following poisons are paired with the correct antidote:**
    A. organophosphates and pralidoxime.
    B. ethylene glycol and methanol.
    C. cyanide and dicobalt edetate.
    D. lead and dimercaprol.
    E. digoxin and Fab antibodies.

18. **AE**

The blood–brain barrier is effectively the endothelium of the cerebral capillaries. Like the passage of drugs across any membrane, transfer is related to size, protein binding and lipid solubility. Only oxygen, carbon dioxide and water enter the brain with ease, and there are transport systems for glucose, amino acids and potassium. The anticholinergics atropine and hyoscine readily cross the blood–brain barrier but glycopyrrolate, because of its quaternary ammonium structure, does not. Benzylpenicillin normally crosses the blood–brain barrier very poorly, except when this is damaged (e.g. in meningitis) when it crosses more readily. In general, muscle relaxants and anticholinesterases do not cross the blood–brain barrier, the exception being physostigmine which is therefore used to treat the central cholinergic syndrome.

19. **AB**

All adverse drug reactions to new drugs (identified by a black triangle in the British National Formulary) and serious or unusual reactions to established drugs should be reported using the CSM yellow card system. These cards are found in the back of the British National Formulary and should be completed as fully as possible and sent by Freepost to the CSM. Drugs used in clinical trials will be reported directly by the trial organizers.

20. **ACE**

Poison	Antidote
Organophosphate	Atropine and pralidoxime
Ethylene glycol or methanol	Ethanol
Cyanide	Dicobalt edetate
Lead	Penicillamine
Arsenic	Dimercaprol
Thallium	Prussian blue
Digoxin	Fab antibodies

21. **Enoximone:**
   A. increases myocardial intracellular cAMP levels.
   B. causes a rise in systemic vascular resistance.
   C. is an imidazolone derivative.
   D. activates phosphodiesterase.
   E. causes an increase in cardiac output.

22. **Solutions of hydroxyethyl heta starch:**
   A. cause a greater increase in plasma volume than the volume infused.
   B. have a similar average molecular weight to albumin.
   C. are partly cleared by the reticuloendothelial system.
   D. have a pH in the range 5.0–5.5.
   E. may affect clotting mechanisms if given in large volumes.

23. **Drugs which are metabolized mainly by esterases include:**
   A. mivacurium.
   B. remifentanil.
   C. atracurium.
   D. cocaine.
   E. lignocaine.

21. ACE

Enoximone is an imidazolone derivative that acts by inhibiting phosphodiesterase and so causes a rise in intracellular cAMP. The increase in cardiac output is due to an increase in stroke volume and a reduction in systemic vascular resistance and it is particularly useful in congestive heart failure. Dosage is by loading dose of 90 µg/kg followed by 5–20 µg/kg per min, but the drug cannot be infused through glass apparatus because a reaction occurs resulting in the formation of crystals. Adverse effects of enoximone include arrhythmias, hypotension, nausea and vomiting, headaches and diarrhoea.

22. ACDE

Solutions of hydroxyethyl heta starch consist of 90% amylopectin etherified with hydroxyethyl groups and have a high average molecular weight (450 000 daltons) compared with that of albumin (67 000 daltons). This accounts for the very slow elimination of these products from the body, which is by liver metabolism and renal excretion. When more than 1000 ml is administered to an adult there may be interference with clotting mechanisms.

23. ABD

Drugs mainly metabolized by esterases include the following:

Cocaine
Amethocaine
Prilocacine
Diamorphine
Esmolol
Mivacurium
Remafentanil.

24. **The following drugs induce liver enzymes:**
    A. chronic administration of phenytoin.
    B. cimetidine.
    C. rifampicin.
    D. carbamazepine.
    E. propranolol.

25. **The following drugs are liver enzyme inhibitors:**
    A. cimetidine.
    B. isoniazid.
    C. warfarin.
    D. sodium valproate.
    E. metronidazole.

26. **The following drugs may cause hepatocellular jaundice:**
    A. isoniazid.
    B. halothane.
    C. methysergide.
    D. chlorpromazine.
    E. paracetamol.

24. ACD

Enzyme induction refers to an absolute increase in enzyme amount and activity due to exposure to a particular drug or chemical and is accompanied by hypertrophy of liver cell endoplasmic reticulum, which contains most drug-metabolizing enzymes. Enzyme inducers share some common properties: they are lipid soluble, substrates for the enzymes that they induce and have a relatively long half-life. Examples of liver-enzyme inducers include barbiturates, carbamazepine, griseofulvin, ethanol, phenytoin, progesterone, rifampicin, glutethimide and DDT.

26. ABDE

Enzyme inhibition of drug metabolism is important because raised levels of the active drug may cause excessive effects, although enzyme inhibition tends to be more selective than enzyme induction. Examples of enzyme inhibition include those listed in the table.

Drug	Inhibits metabolism of
Cimetidine	Propranolol
Allopurinol	Azathioprine
Isoniazid	Phenytoin
Sodium valproate	Phenytoin
Metronidazole	Ethanol

26. BE

Drug causes of jaundice may be classified as listed in the table.

Prehepatic
Drugs that cause haemolysis, e.g. hydralazine
Hepatic
Halothane (and other volatile anaesthetic agents)
Paracetamol
Methotrexate
Post-hepatic
Chlorpromazine
Erythromycin
Methysergide (may cause a posthepatic jaundice as a secondary effect of sclerosing cholangitis)

27. Ephedrine:
- **A.** may be given by the intramuscular route.
- **B.** is a bronchodilator.
- **C.** has β_1-adrenergic agonist effects.
- **D.** may cause cardiac arrhythmias.
- **E.** maintains placental blood flow.

28. Pancuronium:
- **A.** is a steroid.
- **B.** has a vagotonic action.
- **C.** blocks sympathetic ganglia.
- **D.** is contraindicated for use during Caesarean section.
- **E.** may cause a reduction in prothrombin time.

29. The following drugs cause uterine relaxation:
- **A.** salbutamol.
- **B.** nifedipine.
- **C.** aminophylline.
- **D.** prostaglandin $F_{2\alpha}$.
- **E.** vecuronium.

30. Pethidine:
- **A.** is synthetic.
- **B.** is more potent than morphine.
- **C.** causes less constipation than morphine.
- **D.** is available as an oral preparation.
- **E.** is metabolized to an active compound.

27. ABCDE

Ephedrine has several clinical effects, including α-adrenergic and β₁-adrenergic agonist effects, and is useful in the prophylaxis and treatment of hypotension following sympathetic blockade (e.g. during spinal anaesthesia). Although ephedrine is usually administered intravenously, it can be effective via the intramuscular route in an emergency, but care should be exercised in diabetic patients and cardiac arrhythmias may be a side-effect of treatment.

28. AE

Pancuronium is a steroid-based neuromuscular blocking agent that has little ganglion-blocking effect and is vagolytic, which may be an advantage if given in combination with vagotonic opioids such as fentanyl and is a reason it is popularly employed in cardiac anaesthesia. Very high doses may cause a reduction in prothrombin time. Pancuronium has a half-life of 116 min and is initially given as a bolus of 0.1 mg/kg (which acts for approximately 2 hours). It has a volume of distribution of 0.31 l/kg and a clearance of 1.8 ml/kg per min.

29. ABC

Uterine relaxation	Uterine contraction
Nifedipine	Oxytocin
Aminophylline	Prostaglandin $F_{2\alpha}$
Magnesium	Ergometrine
Indomethacin	Histamine H_2 agonists
Salbutamol	

30. ACDE

Pethidine is a synthetic opioid that has a potency approximately one-tenth that of morphine. It causes less constipation and histamine release compared with morphine but is less efficacious. It can be given orally as well as intravenously and intramuscularly, but not subcutaneously as it is too irritant. Pethidine has an anticholinergic effect and local anaesthetic action; it does not delay labour in pregnant women, but does cross the placenta. It is metabolized to the active compound, nor-pethidine, which possesses proconvulsant activity.

31. **The following conditions are associated with hyperglycaemia:**
    A. hypothyroidism.
    B. acromegaly.
    C. Cushing's syndrome.
    D. glucagonoma.
    E. haemochromatosis.

32. **Lack of dietary thiamine (vitamin B₁) results in the following:**

    A. heart failure.
    B. anaemia.
    C. pellagra.
    D. Korsakoff's syndrome.
    E. night blindness.

33. **The following are true regarding the limbic system:**
    A. it is formed in part by the amygdala and hippocampus.
    B. it is partly concerned with taste.
    C. the Papez circuit is a closed circuit linking the limbic system with the thalamus.
    D. stimulation produces autonomic effects.
    E. lesions cause anorexia.

34. **Lymphatic fluid contains the following:**
    A. proteins.
    B. clotting factors.
    C. fats.
    D. lymphocytes.
    E. haemoglobin.

31. BCDE

Secondary diabetes (a fasting blood sugar of > 7 mmol/l) may be caused by the following:

acromegaly
Cushing's syndrome
haemochromatosis
thyrotoxicosis
carcinoma of the pancreas
phaeochromocytoma
glucagonoma
drugs, such as steroids and thiazide diuretics.

32. AD

Thiamine is a coenzyme in carboxylase, the enzyme necessary for carbohydrate metabolism; relative deficiency is common in alcoholics (who have a high carbohydrate intake due to the alcohol) and is associated with heart failure (beri beri) and the Korsakoff syndrome (retrograde amnesia, confabulation, lack of insight, diminished drive and apathy). Deficiency is diagnosed by a reduction in red blood cell transketolase activity. Anaemia is due to folic acid or vitamin B_{12} deficiency, whilst pellagra occurs in niacin deficiency and night blindness is due to vitamin A deficiency.

33. ABCD

The limbic system is formed by the hippocampus, amygdala and septal nuclei, and its functions include olfaction, feeding, sexual behaviour and the emotions of fear and rage. Stimulation produces autonomic effects (indicating higher cortical connections) as well as chewing and licking motions, whilst lesions within the limbic system result in hyperphagia rather than anorexia.

34. ABCD

Lymphatic fluid contains protein (although in lower concentrations than in the plasma), clotting factors (and will therefore clot if left to stand), lymphocytes and fats (causing lymphatic fluid to appear cloudy after a meal). Lymphatic fluid drains via the right lymphatic duct and the thoracic duct on the left into the superior vena cava.

35. **The following are true regarding immunoglobulins:**
    A. IgM is the immunoglobulin found in the highest concentrations within the circulation.
    B. the basic immunoglobulin unit consists of four polypeptide chains.
    C. there are two types of light chain and two types of heavy chain.
    D. lymphocytes secrete immunoglobulins.
    E. IgE causes histamine release from basophils and mast cells.

36. **The following are correct regarding the aqueous humour of the eye:**
    A. it is produced by the retinal blood vessels.
    B. it is reabsorbed into the canal of Schlemm.
    C. it is produced at the rate of approximately 1 ml/min.
    D. it fills the space between the lens and the retina.
    E. obstruction of its drainage results in glaucoma.

37. **The following are true regarding serotonin (5HT):**
    A. the highest concentrations are found in the gastrointestinal tract and within platelets.
    B. it is formed from dietary tryptophan.
    C. it is metabolized by serotonin peptase.
    D. its urinary metabolite is vanillylmandelic acid (VMA).
    E. in the pineal gland it is converted to melatonin.

38. **Administration of growth hormone results in an increase in the following:**
    A. erythropoiesis.
    B. 2,3-diphosphoglycerate (2,3-DPG).
    C. calcium absorption from the gastrointestinal tract.
    D. free fatty acid utilization.
    E. insulin release from the pancreas.

39. **The following are true of nerves:**
    A. pain and temperature sensation are transmitted via Aδ and B fibres.
    B. somatic motor nerves are B fibres.
    C. postganglionic sympathetic nerves are C fibres.
    D. touch sensation is transmitted via Aα and Aδ fibres.
    E. preganglionic autonomic nerves are B fibres.

35. **BE**

Of the five different immunoglobulins, IgG is found in the highest concentration (constituting 75% of circulating immunoglobulins whereas IgA constitutes 20% and IgM 5%). The basic component of immunoglobulins are four polypeptide chains (two light and two heavy chains) and there are two types of light chains and five types of heavy chains. Immunoglobulins are secreted by plasma cells.

36. **BCE**

Aqueous humour is a clear fluid produced by the ciliary body (by diffusion and active transport) and is reabsorbed into the canal of Schlemm. It is the viscous vitreous humour that fills the posterior chamber between the lens and the retina.

37. **ABE**

Serotonin is formed by the hydroxylation and decarboxylation of dietary tryptophan, and is found in highest concentrations in platelets and the enterochromaffin cells and myenteric plexus of the gastrointestinal tract. There are at least five different serotonin receptors; e.g. stimulation of $5HT_2$ receptors results in platelet aggregation and smooth muscle contraction. Serotonin is metabolized by monoamine oxidase to the urinary metabolite 5-hydroxyindole acetic acid (5-HIAA) and raised levels of this are found in patients with carcinoid syndrome.

38. **ABCD**

Growth hormone is an anabolic hormone causing an increase in metabolic rate, increased calcium absorption from the gastro-intestinal tract, and a reduction in the renal excretion of sodium and potassium. Growth hormone causes an increase in erythro-poietin and 2,3-DPG production and has an anti-insulin effect.

39. **CDE**

	Diameter (µm)	Velocity (m/s)
Aα Somatic motor and proprioception	12–20	70–120
Aβ Touch and pressure	5–12	30–70
Aγ Motor to muscle spindles	3–6	15–30
Aδ Pain and temperature	2–5	12–30
B Preganglionic autonomic	< 3	3–15
C Postganglionic sympathetic and dorsal root pain and temperature	0.3–1.3	0.5–2

40. When an aircraft is flying at cruising altitude of 35 000 feet:
- **A.** a small pneumothorax may develop into a tension pneumothorax.
- **B.** arterial oxygen saturation may drop by 5%.
- **C.** females with an uncomplicated pregnancy may fly until 36 weeks' gestation.
- **D.** patients should not fly 6 weeks after an uncomplicated myocardial infarction.
- **E.** commercial airlines routinely provide high-flow oxygen for emergency purposes.

41. The following are polysynaptic reflexes:
- **A.** withdrawal.
- **B.** abdominal.
- **C.** knee.
- **D.** cremasteric.
- **E.** inverse stretch.

42. Regarding light sensors in the eye:
- **A.** rods detect light at night-time.
- **B.** rods are especially concentrated on the macula.
- **C.** there are two types of cones.
- **D.** colour blindness is detected clinically by the use of Ishihara charts.
- **E.** at dusk there is a change from colour to monochromatic sight.

40.   ABC

Most commercial aircraft fly at an altitude of around 35 000 feet and have a cabin pressure equivalent to flying at an altitude of around 7000 feet. The partial pressure of arterial oxygen may drop from 13.3 kPa to about 10.3 kPa and the arterial oxygen saturation by between 3 and 10%. Gases within body cavities may expand in volume by up to 30%: a small pneumothorax may become a tension pneumothorax, middle ear problems may occur and gas within the intestinal lumen may cause tension on suture lines if recent surgery has been performed. There is an increased risk of deep vein thrombosis due to relative immobility during 'long-haul' flights. Commercial airlines provide portable low-flow oxygen from cylinders and carry Hudson masks. Most airlines recommend that the following customers should not fly:

within 10 days of an uncomplicated myocardial infarction
if the serum haemoglobin is less than 7.5 g/dl
if a female is more than 36 weeks pregnant (or into the third
   trimester of a complicated pregnancy)
newborn babies until they are 7 days old.

41.   ABDE

All the above are polysynaptic reflexes except the knee jerk which, together with the ankle, biceps and triceps reflex, is a monosynaptic reflex. Polysynaptic reflex paths branch in a complex fashion. The number of synapses in each of their branches is variable and, because of the synaptic delay incurred at each synapse, activity in the branches with fewer synapses reaches the motor neurones first, followed by activity in the longer pathways. This causes prolonged bombardment of the motor neurones from a single stimulus and consequently prolonged responses. Also, some of the branch pathways turn back on themselves and activity reverberates until the response dies out.

42.   ADE

The rods and cones are specialized sensors on the retina that detect light. There are three types of cones (red, blue and green), which are especially concentrated on the macula and detect light during the daytime. During dusk there is a change from coloured to monochromatic vision when the rods take over sensing light; this change-over takes approximately 30 min and is called the Purkinje shift.

43. **The following are true regarding the ear:**
    A. perilymph has a constitution similar to cerebrospinal fluid (CSF).
    B. the cochlear nerve travels via the internal capsule to the superior temporal gyrus.
    C. the semicircular canals detect linear acceleration.
    D. a whisper produces a sound of approximately 40 dB.
    E. there is a linear increase in sound as measured in the decibel range.

44. **The following are at least partially metabolized in the lung:**
    A. morphine.
    B. prostaglandins.
    C. 5HT (serotonin).
    D. kallikrein.
    E. acetylcholine.

43. **ABD**

   In the ear nerve endings that detect sound are found in the tectorial membrane at the base of hairs. Impulses travel via the cochlear nerve to the superior temporal gyrus (the auditory cortex). Sound is measured in decibels (dB), which is a logarithmic scale; the doubling from 10 to 20 dB indicates a 10-fold increase in noise level; 40 dB is the level of a whisper, whilst 80 dB is traffic level and 120 dB level causes pain. The semicircular canals detect angular acceleration, whilst the otolith organs (modified hairs) detect linear acceleration.

44. **BCE**

   Along with gas exchange, the lungs are capable of the functions listed in the table.

Metabolism	Activation
Prostaglandins	Angiotensin I to angiotensin II
Acetylcholine	**Synthesis**
Noradrenaline	Surfactant
5HT	Prostaglandins
Bradykinin	
Adenine nucleotides	

45. **Surfactant:**
    A. consists of proteins, carbohydrates and fats.
    B. is produced in the liver and lungs.
    C. production is increased if the inspired oxygen concentration is increased.
    D. deficiency results in impaired diffusion of carbon dioxide.
    E. may be synthetically produced.

46. **Normochromic, normocytic anaemia with an increased reticulocyte count occurs in:**
    A. haemorrhage.
    B. secondary malignant deposits in the bone marrow.
    C. haemolysis.
    D. bone marrow aplasia.
    E. vitamin B_{12} deficiency.

45. AE

Surfactant is produced by the type II alveolar cells of the lung and contains fat (90%), protein (8%) and carbohydrate (2%). The main effect of surfactant is to reduce surface tension and thereby the tendency of the alveoli to collapse. There are four surfactant proteins: A and D proteins are large and B and C proteins are small and hydrophobic. Synthesis of surfactant is developmentally regulated in fetal lung and can be accelerated by glucocorticoids and other hormones. The majority of surfactant is removed from the alveolar space by reuptake into the type II cells by mechanisms that include receptor-mediated endocytosis. Some components of surfactant are directly recycled into new surfactant whereas other components are degraded. Production of surfactant is impaired in the following conditions:

> fetal hyperinsulinaemia (this is probably the reason why babies of diabetic mothers are more likely to develop idiopathic respiratory distress syndrome, IRDS)
> hypothyroidism
> exposure to cigarette smoke
> pulmonary circulatory disturbances (e.g. cardiopulmonary bypass, pulmonary embolus)
> bronchial obstruction
> long-term 100% oxygen therapy.

Surfactant may be synthesized, as well as being available from natural sources, e.g. bovine lung.

46. AC

Reticulocytes are red blood cells without a nucleus, but which contain ribosomal RNA and so appear speckled on a blood film. They spend 1–2 days in the bone marrow and then a further 1–2 days in the peripheral blood before maturing (mainly in the spleen), when the RNA is completely lost. Following stimulation of erythropoiesis in acute blood loss (haemorrhage or haemolysis) the reticulocytes are released prematurely from the bone marrow and spend relatively longer in the peripheral circulation and hence a higher number, or percentage, is recorded. Bone marrow secondary deposits and aplasia result in a normochromic, normocytic anaemia, but not a reticulocyte response. Vitamin B_{12} deficiency causes a megaloblastic anaemia.

47. **Oxygen supply to the heart is dependent upon:**
    A. haemoglobin concentration.
    B. blood viscosity.
    C. heart rate.
    D. sympathetic tone.
    E. acidity of the blood.

48. **In Fallot's tetralogy, cyanosis is increased by:**
    A. exercise.
    B. taking a hot bath.
    C. crying.
    D. squatting.
    E. feeding.

47. ABCDE

Assuming that coronary blood flow is laminar, coronary blood flow is proportional to:

(aortic diastolic pressure − LVEDP) × radius^4/viscosity

where LVEDP is left ventricular end-diastolic pressure. Most blood flows during diastole and thus an increase in heart rate reduces the diastolic time as well as increasing oxygen consumption. The radius of the blood vessels is affected by sympathetic tone and local factors such as acidosis, hypoxia and hypercarbia. Oxygen delivery also depends upon the oxygen content of the blood (i.e. the haemoglobin concentration, percentage oxygen saturation and amount of dissolved oxygen).

48. ABCE

Fallot's tetralogy consists of:

    ventriculoseptal defect (VSD)
    pulmonary stenosis
    right ventricular hypertrophy
    over-riding aorta.

There is a right to left shunt and deoxygenated blood enters the systemic circulation, resulting in resting cyanosis. This is made worse when the metabolic rate is increased, e.g. when crying, feeding, taking a bath or exercising. Squatting is a method that children develop to reduce venous return to the right side of the heart and also increase systemic afterload, thereby reducing the amount of right to left shunting and hence cyanosis. Treatment of this condition is usually surgical, although the use of β-adrenergic blockers may lessen the episodes of cyanosis. The initial surgery at a young age consists of creating a shunt between the aorta and the pulmonary artery in order that sufficient blood can enter the lungs; a Blalock shunt is from subclavian artery to pulmonary artery or a Waterston shunt is from ascending aorta to right pulmonary artery. When the child approaches school age total correction of the defects is carried out.

49. One litre of Hartmann's solution (compound sodium lactate) contains:
A. 150 mmol sodium.
B. 135 mmol chloride.
C. 29 mmol lactate.
D. 5 mmol potassium.
E. 5 mmol calcium.

50. Regarding a post-dural puncture headache:
A. it is due to CSF leakage.
B. the administration of intravenous fluids increases the rate of CSF production.
C. an epidural blood patch, if performed, should be sited caudal to the original dural puncture.
D. some of the blood taken to perform a blood patch should be sent for microbiological culture.
E. an epidural blood patch usually relieves the headache immediately.

49. CD

> One litre of Hartmann's solution contains
>   131 mmol of sodium
>   111 mmol of chloride
>   29 mmol of lactate
>   5 mmol of potassium
>   2 mmol of calcium
>
> One litre of normal saline contains
>   150 mmol of sodium
>   150 mmol of chloride
>
> One litre of dextrose saline contains
>   30 mmol of sodium
>   30 mmol of chloride
>   40 g of glucose
>
> One litre of 5% dextrose contains 50 g of glucose

50. ACDE

It is now established that post-dural puncture headaches are due to CSF leakage and, because CSF production is independent of the hydrational status of the patient, intravenous fluids will not affect production of CSF (but may reduce the severity of the headache by improving overall hydration). Epidural blood patches should be performed by a senior anaesthetist and sited caudal to the original dural tap (it has been shown that the majority of blood injected into the epidural space travels cephalad). A second anaesthetist should have aseptically withdrawn approximately 40 ml of venous blood, 20 ml of which is injected through the epidural needle and the rest sent for microbiological culture.

51. **In patients suffering from cystic fibrosis:**
    A. lung bullae may be present.
    B. diabetes mellitus is possible.
    C. regional anaesthesia is contraindicated.
    D. atropine is a good premedicant.
    E. a preoperative ECG should be performed.

52. **Patients with hypothyroidism:**
    A. may present with angina.
    B. are resistant to the effects of fentanyl.
    C. should be given perioperative steroid cover.
    D. are susceptible to intraoperative hypothermia.
    E. should be hyperventilated during anaesthesia.

53. **β_1-Sympathomimetic effects include:**
    A. bronchoconstriction.
    B. piloerection.
    C. increase in renin release.
    D. uterine relaxation.
    E. increase in atrioventricular node conduction.

51.   ABE

Cystic fibrosis is an autosomal recessive condition (with an incidence of 1 in 2000), that is due to an abnormality of chromosome 7 and results in abnormalities of the exocrine glands. Diagnosis is usually made in early childhood by finding a sweat sodium concentration of greater than 30 mmol/l. Respiratory problems include recurrent infections (usually due to *Staphylococcus* or *Pseudomonas*), lung bullae and basal bronchiectasis. Patients may develop right ventricular failure (cor pulmonale) secondary to pulmonary hypertension, as well as malabsorption, diabetes and nasal polyps. Patients take prophylactic antibiotics and pancreatic supplements and, when they present for surgery, preoperative management includes obtaining a chest radiograph and ECG, chest physiotherapy (including postural drainage) and inhaled nebulizers. Drying agents such as atropine should be avoided as secretions are already viscid, and regional anaesthesia is a useful technique to employ in these patients.

52.   AD

Hypothyroidism causes the following clinical features:

> bradycardia and ischaemic heart disease
> weight gain and constipation
> impaired recovery of tendon reflexes, peripheral neuropathy, cerebellar abnormalities and dementia
> gout and menorrhagia
> hair loss, hoarse voice, carpal tunnel syndrome, hearing loss, puffy face, non-pitting oedema and cold intolerance.

Patients are sensitive to central nervous system (CNS) depressants, develop hypothermia quickly, but do not require steroid cover.

53.   CE

All β-adrenergic receptors stimulate adenylate cyclase via G protein–receptor coupling, leading to accumulation of cAMP and activation of cAMP-dependent protein kinases. Typically, β_1 effects result in an increase in heart rate, myocardial contraction, conduction and automaticity, and also an increase in renin release from the juxtaglomerular cells of the kidney; β_2 effects include bronchodilatation, an increase in bronchial secretions and uterine relaxation. Pilomotor muscle contraction is an α_1-agonist effect.

54. Recognized features of untreated acromegaly include:
A. hypertension.
B. dry skin.
C. difficulty with tracheal intubation.
D. hypophosphataemia.
E. glucose intolerance.

55. The following are increased in chronic renal failure:
A. erythropoietin release.
B. gastrin secretion.
C. production of 2,3-DPG.
D. albumin concentration.
E. α_1-acid glycoprotein levels.

54. ACE

Acromegaly is due to excessive secretion of growth hormone after puberty (before puberty gigantism results) and is usually due to an acidophil anterior pituitary tumour (although some cases are due to multiglandular disease). Clinical features include those listed in the table.

Those due to the underlying tumour
Headache and bitemporal hemianopia
Those due to the metabolic effects
Excessive soft tissue growth resulting in a large tongue and potential difficulty with tracheal intubation
Hypertension
Greasy skin and acne
Hyperglycaemia
Arthropathy
Cardiomyopathy
Carpal tunnel syndrome
Ischaemic heart disease

Diagnosis is made by recording excessive serum growth hormone levels by radioimmunoassay (RIA). Treatment includes bromocriptine (50% of patients respond to this, but the size of the tumour is not reduced), radiotherapy and transsphenoidal surgery to remove the tumour.

55. BCE

In chronic renal failure there is an increase in the following:

2,3-DPG which, together with acidosis, results in a shift to the right in the oxygen–haemoglobin dissociation curve
prolactin
uric acid
phosphate
gastrin secretion
α_1-acid glycoprotein, resulting in increased plasma protein binding of drugs such as bupivacaine
triglyceride levels.

There is anaemia and impaired platelet function, reduction in erythropoietin release and lowered serum albumin and thyroid binding globulin levels.

56. **In oliguria postoperatively, acute renal failure is compatible with:**
    A. urinary sodium concentration of 10 mmol/l.
    B. urine specific gravity of 1.024.
    C. epithelial casts in the urine.
    D. a serum potassium concentration of 6.7 mmol/l.
    E. urinary urea concentration above the normal range.

57. **The following are associated with angiotensin II:**
    A. most of its effects are caused by binding to type 1 receptors.
    B. thirst.
    C. vasopressin (ADH) release.
    D. renal sodium loss.
    E. its effects are blocked by losartan potassium.

56. CD

Normal values for urinary constituents are shown in the table.

	mmol/day
Sodium	100–250
Potassium	40–100
Urea	300–500
Chloride	150–200
Calcium	2.5–7.5
Creatinine	9–18

Acute renal failure is characterized by inability to concentrate the urine (whose volume is less than 400 ml per 24 hours in adults), excrete urea or retain sodium. This results in the following:

> urine specific gravity of 1.010
> urinary sodium > 30 mmol/l
> urinary urea < 150 mmol/l
> urinary osmolality < 300 mosmol/l
> urine:plasma urea ratio < 4
> urine:plasma osmolality ratio 1.1.

57. ABCE

Angiotensin II exerts effects via type 1 receptors; type 2 receptors are present in the cerebellum and adrenal medulla but their role has not been elucidated. Losartan potassium is a competitive antagonist at type 1 receptors and blocks all known effects of angiotensin II. These effects include:

> vasoconstriction
> renal sodium retention
> aldosterone release
> vasopressin (ADH) release
> thirst
> positive inotropic effect on the heart
> catecholamine release from the adrenal medulla.

58. Regarding epilepsy in pregnancy:

    A. seizures are less likely to occur than in the non-pregnant state.

    B. there is a 10-fold increase in fetal abnormalities in epileptic patients compared with normal pregnancy.

    C. use of sodum valproate during pregnancy is associated with fetal neural tube abnormalities.

    D. use of phenytoin during pregnancy is associated with the fetal hydantoin syndrome.

    E. pregnant patients with treated epilepsy are more likely to bleed excessively during Caesarean section.

58. CD

Epileptic patients on treatment who become pregnant (possibly because anticonvulsants increase the metabolism of oral contraceptive pills) have an even chance of the fits becoming more frequent, less frequent or remaining the same during pregnancy; it is also important that other causes such as eclampsia are ruled out. In patients with no history of fitting, a first convulsion in pregnancy may be a sign of an intracranial lesion (such as a meningioma, arteriovenous malformation or venous thrombosis) and magnetic resonance imaging (MRI) should be performed. The pharmacokinetic changes of anti-convulsants when used in pregnancy are:

reduced absorption from the gastrointestinal tract
increased volume of distribution
reduced protein binding
increased clearance.

The overall result is that serum levels of anticonvulsants may be the same, increased or decreased, and patients intending to become pregnant should be monitored carefully and placed on the lowest dose of a single drug able to control the convulsions. The effects of anticonvulsants on the fetus are as follows.

Two-fold increase in fetal abnormalities, including facial clefts (lip and/or palate).
Sodium valproate causes an increase in neural tube defects (all pregnant patients should take folate supplements).
Phenytoin may cause the fetal hydantoin syndrome (cranio-facial abnormalities, mental retardation and limb defects).
Following delivery, there is an increase in the incidence of neonatal bleeding, probably due to inhibition of the enzyme carboxylase resulting in the production of proteins induced by vitamin K absence or antagonism (PIVKAs). This may be prevented by giving the mother oral vitamin K in pregnancy.

Hopkins, A. (1987) Epilepsy and anticonvulsants. In *Prescribing in Pregnancy* (ed. P.C. Rubin), pp. 96–110. BMJ Publishing, London.

59. **A serum potassium concentration of 6.2 mmol/l and serum sodium concentration of 125 mmol/l are compatible with a diagnosis of untreated:**
    A. Addison's disease.
    B. renal failure.
    C. Cushing's syndrome.
    D. dehydration.
    E. diabetic ketoacidosis.

60. **The presence of pathological Q waves in the inferior ECG leads (II, III and aVF) may be due to:**
    A. pulmonary embolus.
    B. Wolff–Parkinson–White syndrome.
    C. inferior myocardial infarction.
    D. left anterior hemiblock conduction abnormality.
    E. pericarditis.

61. **The following are true regarding ionizing radiation:**
    A. a proton has a positive charge.
    B. a proton has a charge of 1 electron.
    C. a positron has a positive, and a less strong negative charge.
    D. an α particle has three positive charges.
    E. β particles do not exist.

59. **ABE**

Addison's disease is glucocorticoid deficiency due to adrenal dysfunction. This was previously seen quite commonly in association with tuberculosis but 70% of cases are now due to an autoimmune adrenalitis in which most of the cortex is lost but the medulla remains intact; antibodies appear to react with the 21-hydroxylase enzyme. The glucocorticoid and mineralo-corticoid deficiency leads to hyponatraemia and hyperkalaemia. In renal failure, hyperkalaemia is common and may be associated with hyponatraemia if renal sodium loss is high. In diabetic ketoacidosis, the serum potassium level at presentation is usually high and the heavy glycosuria will increase renal sodium loss. In Cushing's syndrome the serum potassium level is usually low and in dehydration the serum sodium level is high.

60. **ABC**

Pathological Q waves (i.e. greater than two small squares deep or one small square wide or more than one-quarter the size of the associated R wave) in the inferior leads occurs in the following conditions:

inferior myocardial infarction
Wolff–Parkinson–White syndrome type B
pulmonary embolus
left posterior hemiblock.

Non-pathological Q waves are common in lead III and disappear on deep inspiration.

61. **A**

A proton has a positive charge of 2000 electrons, whilst a positron has a positive charge of 1 electron. An α particle has two positive charges, whilst β particles are electrons.

62 **The partial pressure of oxygen in a gas may be measured by:**
   A. a fuel cell.
   B. a paramagnetic analyser.
   C. infrared absorption spectrophotometry.
   D. a polarographic analyser.
   E. pulse oximetry.

63. **With regard to MRI and computed tomography (CT) head scans:**
   A. the time taken to perform the scans is similar.
   B. the image plane is vertical for MRI but transverse for CT.
   C. MRI is more accurate for diagnosing demyelinating disease.
   D. ionizing radiation is used in CT scanning.
   E. MRI results in less patient discomfort than CT.

64. **The following are approximately equivalent to a pressure of one atmosphere:**
   A. 100 cm H_2O.
   B. 1 bar.
   C. 760 mmHg.
   D. 100 psi (pounds per square inch).
   E. 15 kPa.

62. ABD

Fuel cells are used to measure the partial pressure of oxygen in a gas mixture and consist of a gold cathode and a lead anode in a potassium hydroxide mixture. The cell produces its own voltage so does not require a battery. Because the reaction is temperature sensitive, this must be maintained constant or be compensated for. Oxygen is paramagnetic and in a paramagnetic analyser a small test chamber is suspended in a magnetic field and filled with the gas mixture; the greater the concentration of oxygen the more the chamber moves and this is detected either by displacement of a light beam or by a transducer. The device is calibrated for differing oxygen tensions. Infrared absorption spectrophotometry relies on the principle that gases containing two or more different atoms absorb infrared radiation with peak absorption of different gases occurring at different wavelengths. Carbon dioxide, nitrous oxide and the volatile anaesthetic agents can all be measured in this manner. The polarographic analyser is an oxygen cell whereby oxygen diffuses into an electrolyte solution via a permeable membrane. There is a platinum cathode and a silver/silver chloride anode with a voltage of $0.6\,V$ applied across the electrodes. Oxygen diffuses into the solution at the cathode and is reduced to hydroxyl ions. A current proportional to the oxygen concentration is produced. Pulse oximeters do not measure oxygen tensions but the proportional saturation of oxygenated haemoglobin.

63. CD

CT scanning uses ionizing radiation whereas MRI uses a large magnet, but both use transverse imaging planes. A CT scan is quicker to perform than MRI and is more comfortable for the patient (MRI can cause severe hearing problems and claustrophobia), but MRI is significantly better for diagnosing some abnormal conditions such as intracranial haematomas and demyelinating diseases.

64. BC

1 bar is approximately equivalent to one atmosphere pressure. This is the same as 15 psi, 101 kPa, 760 mmHg or 1000 cmH$_2$O.

65. **A pulmonary artery balloon flotation catheter:**
    A. can measure pulmonary artery wedge pressure.
    B. directly measures systemic vascular resistance.
    C. can be used to measure mixed venous oxygen saturations continuously.
    D. may be inaccurate when tricuspid regurgitation is present.
    E. can cause a pulmonary infarct.

66. **The Wheatstone bridge:**
    A. may be used to measure an unknown resistance.
    B. involves two potential dividers connected to a common supply voltage.
    C. involves the use of four resistors in series.
    D. is insensitive to small changes.
    E. shows a linear relationship between resistance and voltage.

67. **With regard to electrical circuits:**
    A. the power can be calculated from knowledge of the current and the resistance.
    B. the current in a circuit will be the same at all points.
    C. resistors in series are additive.
    D. the current in a circuit is proportional to the potential difference divided by the resistance.
    E. they are governed by Ohm's law.

68. **The following are true regarding anaesthetic gas cylinders:**
    A. they are made from molybdenum steel.
    B. they must be hydraulically tested every 5 years.
    C. the tare weight is the weight of the full cylinder.
    D. an E size oxygen cylinder contains 680 l when full.
    E. the filling ratio is the weight of substance a cylinder holds divided by the maximum weight that it could hold.

65. ACE

A pulmonary artery balloon flotation catheter (PAFC) or Swan–Ganz catheter can be used to obtain the following information:

pulmonary artery wedge pressure
pulmonary artery pressures
mixed venous oxygen saturations
core temperature
cardiac output using the thermodilution principle
insert pacing wires.

Systemic vascular resistance is one of the many variables that can be derived.

66. AB

The Wheatstone bridge is a circuit consisting of two potential dividers with a common supply voltage. There are four resistors and a voltmeter between the two potential dividers. If the four resistances are equal the voltmeter will not register. If one of the resistances is changed the voltage balance will be altered and this will register as a change in voltage. The relationship is non-linear but is very sensitive to even small changes in voltage.

67. ABCDE

Electrical circuits are governed by Ohm's law, which states that the potential difference (V) is the current (I) multiplied by the resistance (R): $V = IR$. The power (W) can be calculated from the current multiplied by the potential difference: $W = VI$. When resistances are in series they are additive: $R_t = R_1 + R_2$. Resistances in parallel are given by the formula: $1/R_t = 1/R_1 + 1/R_2$.

68. ABD

The tare weight is the weight of the empty cylinder. The plastic ring around the neck of the cylinder indicates when the cylinder was last hydraulically tested (oxygen is tested to a pressure of 3000 psi or 200 atmospheres). The filling ratio is the weight of the full cylinder divided by the weight of the cylinder if it was full of water (in the UK the filling ratio of nitrous oxide is 0.75). When a cylinder full of gas is switched on the pressure indicates the amount remaining; however, in the case of liquids the pressure will not start to drop until the cylinder is nearly empty, and the only way of knowing how much is left is to weigh the cylinder and use knowledge of the tare weight and density of the contents to calculate the volume remaining.

69. **With regard to laryngoscope blades:**
    A. a 'left-handed' blade is available.
    B. the polio blade has an extended angle between the blade and handle.
    C. the Miller blade is appropriate for use in infants.
    D. Macintosh blades are available in three sizes.
    E. Magill blades are curved.

70. **Regarding tracheal tubes:**
    A. single-use disposable tubes have been sterilized before packaging in an autoclave.
    B. standard endotracheal tubes usually have a left-facing bevel.
    C. RAE is an acronym for right angle exit tube.
    D. tracheostomy tubes have a right-facing bevel.
    E. metal tracheostomy tubes are usually made of silver.

71. **The following are true regarding a train-of-four stimulus:**
    A. the response to a single supramaximal stimulus is half the control when 50% of receptors are occupied.
    B. the response to a single supramaximal stimulus is only absent when all the receptors are occupied.
    C. during a train-of-four stimulus, a T2 response reappears when the T1 response returns to approximately 25% of control.
    D. when the T4:T1 ratio is greater than 75%, good muscular tone is usually present.
    E. in normal neuromuscular transmission, post-tetanic potentiation occurs.

69. ABC

Macintosh laryngoscope blades are available in four sizes and are curved, whereas Magill blades are straight. A left-sided Macintosh blade is available for lesions in the right side of the mouth, and a polio blade may be useful in some circumstances. The McCoy laryngoscope consists of a hinged tip operated by a level mechanism present on the handle and may convert a Cormack and Lehane grade 2 or 3 laryngoscopy to a grade 1 or 2 view respectively.

70. BE

Most single-use endotracheal (ET) tubes are implantation tested on rabbits; a small amount from a batch of tubes is injected into the back and the rabbits are sacrificed at 6 weeks and examined for deleterious effects due to plasticizers and dyes. The tubes are sterilized by ethylene oxide. Most ET tubes have a left-facing bevel (to obtain a better view of the vocal cords during insertion) and may have a Murphy eye. There are usually no bevels on tracheostomy tubes. RAE is an acronym for Ring, Adair, Elwin.

71. DE

When a neuromuscular blocking drug is administered, as more receptors at the neuromuscular junction become occupied, the response to a single supramaximal stimulus becomes less as compared with a control response; however, the response is not directly proportional to the percentage of receptors occupied; the clinical response does not start to diminish until approximately 75% of the receptors are occupied, and is absent when approximately 90% of the receptors are occupied. During recovery from neuromuscular blockade the train-of-four response is not directly proportional to receptor occupancy; during a train-of-four stimulus, after the first response reappears, a T2 response appears when the T1 response is 10% of control height, a T3 response appears when the T1 is 20% of control and T4 appears at 50% recovery. This means that all four twitches in a train of four reappear at only 50% recovery from neuromuscular block, but good muscle tone is not restored until 75% recovery has taken place.

72. **In patients with cardiac pacemakers:**
    A. use of diathermy is absolutely contraindicated.
    B. halothane may reduce the threshold for arrhythmias.
    C. suxamethonium should be avoided if possible.
    D. the diathermy earthing plate should be placed as close to the pacemaker as possible.
    E. use of diathermy may damage the pacemaker mechanism.

73. **The following are correct pin index configurations:**
    A. oxygen: 2 and 6.
    B. nitrous oxide: 3 and 5.
    C. Entonox: 3 and 6.
    D. carbon dioxide: 1 and 6.
    E. helium: 2 and 5.

72. **BCE**

Patients fitted with permanent cardiac pacemakers should be assessed preoperatively and the following questions answered.

When was the pacemaker inserted?
Why was the pacemaker inserted?
Has the pacemaker been checked recently?
What type of pacemaker has been fitted and is it working correctly?
Is the patient pacemaker dependent?

At the very least the patient should have a chest radiograph, ECG and electrolytes checked and a cardiologist consulted for advice. Intraoperatively, atropine, isoprenaline, defibrillator machine and temporary pacing leads should be close to hand. Bipolar diathermy use is preferable, but if monopolar diathermy is used the earthing plate should be placed as far away from the pacemaker as possible, and there is a risk of microshock through the pacemaker leads resulting in endocardial burns and reprogramming of the pacemaker. Suxamethonium should be avoided as the fasciculations that occur may be sensed as complexes and cause pacemaker inhibition. Halothane reduces the threshold for cardiac arrhythmias.

73. **BD**

The pin index system was devised in order to prevent the accidental fitting of a cylinder of the wrong gas to a yoke, thus making interchangeability of cylinders of different gases impossible. One or more pins project from the yoke and these locate in holes bored into the valve block of the cylinder. The configuration of the pins varies with each gas and if the wrong cylinder is offered up to the yoke it is impossible to fit. The following are correct pin index configurations:

oxygen: 2 and 5
nitrous oxide: 3 and 5
Entonox: a single pin
carbon dioxide: 1 and 6
helium: no pin index
cyclopropane (when it was in use): 3 and 6.

74. **The following are true with regard to the paediatric Ayres T-piece with Jackson Rees modification:**
    A. it is more efficient for spontaneous compared with positive pressure ventilation.
    B. the expiratory limb should have a volume at least equal to the tidal volume to avoid entrainment of room air.
    C. the fresh gas flow rate during spontaneous breathing must equal the peak inspiratory flow rate.
    D. movement of the reservoir bag is a good indicator of tidal volume.
    E. scavenging waste anaesthetic gases is easy.

75. **The following are true with regard to heat and moisture exchangers (HMEs):**
    A. they are more efficient at high fresh gas flows than low fresh gas flows.
    B. the greater the dead space, the lower the resistance to breathing.
    C. if they are not changed between cases there is a risk of cross-infection.
    D. all HMEs have a dead space of at least 25 ml.
    E. the heat provided to the inspired gases is mainly derived from the latent heat of water in the expired gases.

74. **B**

The Ayres T-piece with Jackson Rees modification is a simple non-valvular system that is equally efficient during spontaneous and positive pressure ventilation. During spontaneous breathing, the fresh gas flow rate required to avoid rebreathing varies with the size of the patient and the design of the T-piece. If the expiratory limb has a capacity as great as the patient's tidal volume, then a fresh gas flow rate of approximately 2.5 times the patient's minute volume will be adequate. If the expiratory limb capacity is less than the tidal volume then a higher fresh gas flow rate is required and, in the extreme, when the expiratory limb is merely an orifice, then the fresh gas flow rate must equal the peak inspiratory flow rate to avoid entrainment of room air and dilution of anaesthetic gases. During spontaneous breathing the reservoir bag is a useful indicator of respiratory rate, but it is not possible to make an accurate assessment of tidal volume simply by observing the bag.

75. **BCE**

HMEs consist of a chamber containing a screen through which the respiratory gases pass in each direction. The screen may consist of wire mesh, foam, aluminium foil or paper. During exhalation the warm moist expired gases impinge on the screen and the specific heat of the gases, together with the latent heat of the water, warm the screen; during inspiration the relatively dry and cool inspired gases are humidified and warmed as they pass through the screen. One of the problems with HMEs is the increase in dead space, although this is not a problem during positive pressure ventilation as the tidal volume can simply be increased; some HMEs have a dead space of only 10 ml compared with others which have a dead space of 90 ml. Resistance to breathing is another problem; this is least with the high-dead-space HMEs compared with the low-dead-space HMEs, all of which are more efficient at low fresh gas flows. HMEs should be changed after each patient use because of the risk of cross-infection between patients.

76. In the TEC Mk 4 vaporizer:
 A. an anti-tip mechanism is included.
 B. the percentage dial cannot be moved unless the locking lever is engaged.
 C. extension rods prevent the use of more than one vaporizer at a time.
 D. a bimetallic strip is located inside the vaporization chamber.
 E. a temperature-sensitive valve adjusts the splitting ratio.

77. The following are SI units (Système International d'Unités):
 A. hertz
 B. watt
 C. psi
 D. calories
 E. litres

78. Entonox cylinders when used for maternal analgesia:
 A. have a two-stage pressure-demand regulator.
 B. may initially deliver low concentrations of oxygen if the cylinder is stored at sub-zero temperature.
 C. can cause megaloblastic anaemia after prolonged exposure.
 D. can be administered by midwives.
 E. contain compressed gases at a pressure of 13 700 kPa.

79. 'Laser resistant' tracheal tubes:
 A. may have two cuffs.
 B. have a cuff that should be filled with air.
 C. may have a flexible silicone body.
 D. do not withstand the effect of carbon dioxide lasers.
 E. reduce the laser strike to healthy tissues by defocusing the reflected beam.

76. **ABCE**
     The TEC Mk 4 vaporizer has the following features:

     a locking lever so that the vaporizer cannot be turned on
     unless the lever is engaged
     interlocking extension rods so that only one vaporizer can be
     switched on at a time
     the splitting ratio is controlled by a temperature-sensitive
     bimetallic valve situated outside the vaporization chamber
     an anti-tip mechanism.

77. **ABE**
     The following are SI units:

length	metre (m)
capacity	litre (l)
temperature	kelvin (K)
mass	kilogram (kg)
pressure	pascal (Pa)
force	newton (N)
energy	joule (J)
power	watt (W)
frequency	hertz (Hz)

78. **ACDE**
     Entonox is a 50:50 mixture of nitrous oxide and oxygen, is
     suitable as an analgesic and is commonly given to women in
     labour. Patients inspire the mixture through a two-stage
     regulator and then breathe out. If the cylinder is cooled to
     less than 5°C then liquefaction occurs, the two substances
     separate, and initially high concentrations of oxygen are
     delivered and then high concentrations of nitrous oxide as
     the oxygen becomes depleted. Long-term administration of
     nitrous oxide has been shown to cause bone marrow depression
     and megaloblastic anaemia.

79. **ACE**
     Laser-resistant tracheal tubes consist of either a flexible stainless
     steel tube or silicone coated tube with a wire spiral and can
     withstand carbon dioxide lasers. Reflected beams are defocused
     to reduce damage to normal tissue and sometimes have two
     cuffs filled with saline in case the outer one is damaged.

80. **The Clark electrode:**
    A. generates a current proportional to the partial pressure of oxygen.
    B. gives an average of inspired and expired concentrations.
    C. does not require calibration.
    D. has a fast response time.
    E. has a 10-year lifespan.

81. **The Hayek oscillator:**
    A. is a type of cuirass.
    B. requires the patient to be intubated.
    C. is available in three different sizes.
    D. maintains a negative-pressure baseline.
    E. is applied to the chest and abdomen.

82. **The following are true with regard to tracheal tubes:**
    A. an Oxford tube has a bevel facing posteriorly.
    B. uncuffed oral RAE tubes have a single 'Murphy eye'.
    C. reinforced tracheal tubes cannot be cut to the desired length.
    D. microlaryngeal tubes have an internal diameter of 5.5 mm.
    E. standard oral tracheal tubes are implantation tested on rats.

83. **An infrared analyser to measure isoflurane concentration:**
    A. is affected by water vapour.
    B. must be calibrated if other anaesthetic agents are used.
    C. commonly uses wavelengths of 9–12 µm.
    D. contains optical filters.
    E. when used within a circle system can return the sample to the breathing system.

80. **AB**

A Clark electrode consists of an electrode that generates a current proportional to the partial pressure of oxygen. It has a slow response time (about 20 s), gives an average of inspiratory and expiratory concentrations, an accuracy of ± 3%, must be calibrated regularly, and has a limited lifespan (approximately 3 years due to deterioration of the Teflon membrane).

81. **ADE**

The Hayek oscillator is a form of cuirass that can be used on both intubated and non-intubated patients provided they have a clear airway. There are 10 different sizes of jacket available, which are applied over the chest and most of the abdomen. A power unit provides external high-frequency oscillations around a negative-pressure baseline, whereby the pressure within the jacket is decreased to cause inspiration and then increased (although still remaining negative) to cause expiration at high frequencies.

82. **AC**

Uncuffed oral RAE tubes have two eyes, microlaryngeal tubes have an internal diameter of 5 mm, and disposable tracheal tubes are implantation tested on rabbits.

83. **BCDE**

Gases with two or more different atoms may be analysed using infrared absorption, and this is the mechanism by which inhalational anaesthetic agents are analysed. Gases enter a chamber, are exposed to infrared light and absorb light of a waveform specific to that gas. The amount of absorption is proportional to the concentration. Optical filters are used to select the desired wavelengths (usually 9–12 μm), the sample can be returned to the breathing system, and water vapour has no effect on the performance of the analyser.

84. **The following agents are correctly paired with their respective filler tube colours:**
    A. halothane   orange
    B. enflurane   blue
    C. isoflurane   purple
    D. sevoflurane   yellow
    E. desflurane   green

85. **Stimulators used for regional nerve blocks:**
    A. have a positive lead connected to the needle probe.
    B. use a current of approximately 10 mA.
    C. will still function if the patient is paralysed with drugs.
    D. stimulate for approximately 1 s at a time.
    E. can also be used for detection of neuromuscular blockade.

86. **Regarding the electrocardiograph (ECG):**
    A. a silver or silver chloride electrode is employed.
    B. lead V1 is best for detecting arrhythmias.
    C. lead CM5 is best for detecting ischaemia.
    D. lead CB5 is useful during thoracic anaesthesia.
    E. mains interference may be a problem.

87. **A pH electrode:**
    A. can measure urine pH.
    B. contains a reference electrode in contact with potassium chloride solution.
    C. must be calibrated regularly.
    D. contains pH-sensitive glass.
    E. produces an output of 60 mV per pH unit.

84. **CD**

Anaesthetic agents accidentally filled into the wrong vaporizer may produce dangerously high concentrations of that agent, so the Fraser–Sweatman pin safety system was developed. Anaesthetic agents are sold in different types of bottle, and a filler tube for each agent with a cap to fit only the appropriate bottle is used. This filler tube ends in a small block that has a slot cut into it which is unique to that anaesthetic agent. The corresponding vaporizer has a plug that will accept only the appropriate filling tube block. The following agents are correctly paired with their respective filler tube colours:

halothane	red
enfurane	orange
isoflurane	purple
sevoflurane	yellow
desflurane	blue

85. **C**

Nerve stimulators used for regional nerve blocks are different from those used to check neuromuscular blockade. They consist of a negative probe and a positive connected to an ECG electrode attached to the patient. A small (0.25–0.5 mA) current is applied at a frequency of 1–2 Hz for 1–2 ms. The machine will still function if the patient is paralysed, but no response will be seen.

86. **ACDE**

The ECG electrode consists of a silver or silver chloride electrode held in a cup. During anaesthesia three skin electrodes are used: left arm, right arm and an indifferent electrode. Lead II is useful for detecting arrhythmias, whilst lead CM5 (manubrium, V5 and left arm electrodes) detects ischaemia and CB5 (right scapula, V5 and left arm electrodes) is a good lead for thoracic anaesthesia. Mains interference of 50 Mh_z, or diathermy, can cause fuzziness of the ECG.

87. **ABCDE**

A pH electrode contains a silver or silver chloride electrode placed in a buffer solution surrounded by a pH-sensitive glass bulb, and a reference electrode of mercury. A pH gradient exists between the test solution and the buffer, which results in an electrical potential of approximately 60 mV per unit pH. It must be calibrated regularly and kept at a constant temperature.

88. **The Manley Servovent ventilator:**
    A. is a minute volume divider.
    B. is driven by the fresh gas flow.
    C. cannot be used with a circle system.
    D. has a tidal volume control knob.
    E. must contain a bacterial filter as some of the components cannot be sterilized.

89. **A Boyle's bottle:**
    A. is available in one size only.
    B. is temperature compensated.
    C. is calibrated from 0 to 10%.
    D. has all the fresh gas passing through it when fully on.
    E. may be used with desflurane.

90. **The following are true with regard to intravenous fluids and giving sets:**
    A. the standard blood filter used is 40-μm mesh size.
    B. the standard giving set is 4 mm internal diameter.
    C. 1 ml of blood is equivalent to 15 drops.
    D. in the paediatric burette 1 ml is equivalent to 60 drops of clear fluid.
    E. clear fluids flow at 200 ml/min through an 18-G cannula.

88. DE

The Manley Servovent ventilator is a bag squeezer, the driving gas is compressed air or oxygen under pressure. There are on–off, inspiratory flow rate control and expiratory time knobs, the machine can be used with a circle system, and part of the equipment is not detachable for sterilization.

89. D

The Boyle's bottle was commonly used in the past to vaporize ether, methoxyflurane and trichloroethylene and is not temperature compensated or calibrated. When the lever is in the off position, none of the fresh gas passes through the vaporizer, but when in the fully on position all the fresh gas passes through the vaporizer. Two sizes of bottle are used, a broad one for ether and a narrow one for other vapours. The concentration of the vapour depends on the temperature, the level of the liquid agent in the bottle and the fresh gas flow rate.

90. BCD

Standard blood-giving sets have an internal diameter of 4 mm and a filter of 150 μm, and blood drops through the reservoir in a volume equivalent to 15 drops per ml (clear fluids are 20 drops per ml). The paediatric burette has 60 drops of clear fluid being equivalent to 1 ml. If distilled water at 22°C under a pressure of 10 kPa flows through tubing 4 mm in diameter and 110 cm long, the following flow rates are achieved with the different-sized cannulae:

20G	50 ml/min
18G	100 ml/min
16G	150 ml/min
14G	300 ml/min

Index

Intracellular fluid 125, 126
Intravascular space 119, 120
Intravenous administration 119, 120
Intravenous fluids 299, 300
Intubating fibrescopes 231, 232
Ionization 27, 28
Ionizing radiation 281, 282
Isoflurane 13, 14, 179, 247, 248
  infrared analyser 295, 296
Isomeric forms 181, 182
  stereoisomers 193, 194
Isoniazid 255, 256

Jackson Rees modification 291, 292
Jaundice, drug-induced 256
Jugular venous pulse (JVP) 121, 122

Ketamine 107, 108, 114, 253, 254

L-dopa 117, 118
Lack circuit 163, 164
Lambert-Beer law 73, 74
Laminar flow 59, 60
Laryngeal mask airway (LMA) 227, 228, 231, 232
Laryngoscope blades 287, 288
Laser resistant tracheal tubes 293, 294
Lasers 223, 224
Laudanosine 3, 4
Lignocaine 11, 12, 17, 18, 111, 112, 241, 242
Limbic system 259, 260
Lithotomy position 79, 80
Liver enzyme inhibition 255, 256
Liver failure, respiratory changes 131, 132
Liver synthetic activity
  enzyme induction 255, 256
  liver disease 131, 132
Losartan 117, 118
Low molecular weight heparins 107, 108
Lower oesophageal barrier pressure 101, 102
Lung metabolic functions 265, 266
Lymphatic fluid 259, 260

Magill breathing system 157, 158
Magnesium 125, 126

Magnetic resonance imaging (MRI)
  head scan 283, 284
  monitoring during 85, 86
Manley MP3 ventilator 233, 234
Manley Servovent ventilator 299, 300
Mapleson D breathing systems 65, 66
Metabolic acidosis 53, 54
Methaemoglobinuria 77, 78
Methohexitone 114, 189, 190
Metoclopramide 245, 246, 249, 250
Metronidazole 245, 246, 255, 256
Microcirculation 211, 212
Midazolam 111, 112, 241, 242
Mivacurium 239, 240, 254
Mixed venous oxygen saturation 31, 32
Monitoring requirements 73, 74
Monoamine oxidase inhibitors (MAOIs) 197, 198
Morphine 23, 24
Muscarinic receptors 241, 242
Myocardial contractility 57, 58
Myocardial muscle 123, 124

Nasal cannulae 227, 228
Needle valves 235, 236
Neonatal physiology 137, 138
Neostigmine 101, 102, 253, 254
Nephrotoxic drugs 187, 188
Nerve physiology 261, 262
Neuromuscular blockade
  drug interactions 5, 6
  residual blockade assessment 75, 76
Nifedipine 5, 8
Nitric oxide (NO) 91, 92
Nitrous oxide 14, 153, 154
  pipeline delivery 225, 226
Noradrenaline reuptake inhibitors 95, 96

Obese patients 49, 50
Oliguria, postoperative 277, 278
Omeprazole 189, 190
Ondansetron 197, 198
One-lung ventilation 51, 52
Opioid receptors 24, 241, 242
Opioids, epidural 115, 116
Oral bioavailability 11, 12
Osmotic diuretics 7, 8, 93, 94

Acids - Ionised Above pH pka

Bases - Ionised Below pH pka

Printed in the United Kingdom
by Lightning Source UK Ltd.
121236UK00001B/578

9 780702 021602